CONQUER HASHIMOTO'S

How to Achieve Remission from Autoimmune Disease, Shrink Thyroid Nodules, and Avoid Surgery

Julie A. Diaz, CHC

First published by Ultimate World Publishing 2024
Copyright © 2024 Julie Diaz

ISBN

Paperback: 978-1-923123-78-6
Ebook: 978-1-923123-79-3

Cover design: Karin Hansen
Layout and typesetting: Ultimate World Publishing
Editor: Marinda Wilkinson

Ultimate World Publishing
Diamond Creek,
Victoria Australia 3089
www.writeabook.com.au

ULTIMATE WORLD
PUBLISHING

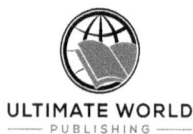

Testimonials

I truly love the story of Julie and her love for her mom. This book exudes Julie's passion to help others. She describes examples of her many medical issues, her course work, and the medical mistakes she suffered during her journey for health. Julie brilliantly and humbly uses these private moments to help others. The book is a page-turner beginning with the most heartwarming dedication. This book will teach the reader about nutrient deficiencies, how to identify the root causes of disease, and the importance of detoxification. Julie, in a very easy to understand way, explains fascinating healing techniques not used in conventional medicine. I can't wait for her next book.

Dr Kerry Gelb, Optometric Physician, Host of Open Your Eyes Podcast, Creator of Open your Eyes Documentary

I've been Julie's massage therapist for over 10 years. She first introduced herself to me as a Health Coach and I began following her on social media. I've always been impressed with her desire to educate and inform. She is truly a fountain of information, having done an extensive amount of research on supplements, nutrition, and alternative medicine. During our sessions, there has always been a healthy exchange of information. I usually try to remember at least three "gems of wisdom" or takeaways from every session. It's good that we have dedicated authors like Julie to champion and help us fight the battles on our journey to wellness. As a sidenote, I've always been a big fan of her Indigo Healing Oils product line, especially Lotus body butter. She actually takes the time to infuse the products with crystal energy.

I frequently promote them to my clients, which I believe are some of the finest essential oil-based home remedies available on the market. Good luck with all your endeavors Julie. You are definitely one of the bright stars in our universe trying to make the world a better place.

Bob Grieza, Massage Therapist, Woodbridge, NJ

Julie has spent decades expanding her knowledge and understanding of the root causes of autoimmune disease and the power of integrative medicine to heal, and in this highly accessible and insightful book she explains how we can take control of our health and feel good again. Julie shares her story with honesty and humor, and has inspired me to actively manage my own health and to look at the bigger picture of what is really going on. As someone who has experienced thyroid nodules and surgery, I only wish I had found her book sooner.

Marinda Wilkinson, Writer and Editor, Melbourne, AU

Julie has been a patient of mine for about 15 years. During our visits, we always engage in great conversations about health and wellness. She has a true passion for natural health and sharing her knowledge with others. I'm very proud of her for writing this book and happy to be included in it. Julie has reached remission with Hashimoto's by addressing the root causes and taking the steps she describes in her wonderful book, *Conquer Hashimoto's*. I am sure this book will help a lot of people.

Dr. Cesar B. Holgado, MD, Edison, NJ

Wow! I absolutely love this book. Julie writes about her personal journey and how she healed herself. I found myself laughing at her stories as she talks about how she took matters into her own hands and refused to give up. This book inspired me to take control of my health. Julie amazed me with the amount of detailed information she provides, covering all sorts of illnesses, and just plain wellness. She not only provides a deep dive on thyroid disease, she shows you how get to the root of what causes many illnesses, and explains how to resolve root causes such as viruses, heavy metals, parasites, and gut infections. She also includes many holistic healing methods and great tips for taking control of your health. I would definitely recommend people read *Conquer Hashimoto's* because I now have so much valuable information at my fingertips, and I didn't have to do any of the work! I found myself adding tabs to flag the pages that I want to go back to. This is one book I must share with others because the gift of health is invaluable.

Christa Roseborsky, Author and Nutrition Manager, Ontario, Canada

Julie has lived with disease. She researches disease intensively, and has now written this book on how she regained her health and vitality. It takes a certain type of individual to accomplish this. It takes an even more unique human to write on it so that others may benefit from the endless research hours, endless questions unanswered by traditional doctors and medicine, and endless daily struggle with symptoms, in order to share the answers so that we may benefit from Julie's journey.

Knowing the root cause is gold. Traditional western medicine treats the symptoms rather than getting to the core of the issue. Rather than continuing to damage ourselves unknowingly with dietary and environmental factors that harm us, we can learn and change today by either adding or subtracting culprits on our road to healing and wellness. Julie is a co-pilot on our own path who writes with authority and empathy as a mother who has achieved what most doctors called unachievable (without RX medicines that serve to create of you a cash cow at your local pharmacy). Her success with reversing Hashimoto's naturally, despite the naysayers, shows her steadfast commitment to finding answers. Thanks to Julie's desire to help others, we too can become wellness warriors in our own lives.

Rosamaria Sagastume, MS Survivor, Middletown, NJ

I have been blessed to know Julie for 16 years. We met when we worked together in an IT documentation department. She was a lead technical writer. It didn't take long for me to wonder why she was doing that type of job because she was always researching health issues and solutions. Literally every time I would tell her about a health issue affecting me or my family, she would instantly give me suggestions for supplements or practices to help with our problems, and if by chance she didn't know the answer, she would research and get back to me. She guided me while I cared for my father who had pancreatic cancer and now, she is helping me with my mother's health issues.

She knows so much about so many things from supplements, flower essences, and essential oils to what tests you should ask your doctor for if you're having certain issues. Julie is an amazing person who is so giving of her knowledge. All she wants to do is support and help people. I'm so proud of her for writing her first book and I know it will help so many people because she's very thorough. There's going to be so much information about so many different things. I think people are going to be waiting for her next book to come out!

Karin Hansen, Designer, Surprise, AZ

I reconnected with Julie through a dear friend of ours to help in my journey to heal an autoimmune disorder. Her knowledge and guidance put me on a path of healing with amazing results. I am very excited to read this book and hear what words of wisdom she has to pass on. Thank you Julie !!

Kathy Steinbaum, HR Director, New Jersey

I hired Julie as my health coach. She recommended some amazing supplements that made a tremendous difference in my health! I look forward to learning much more in her book!

Kim Wright, HR Manager, New York

Dedication

I dedicate this book to my mother. Tragically, she died from Covid-19 on April 23, 2020. She was 84 years old. No one should have to die alone and especially not my mother. She deserved so much better. After being orphaned and suffering many hardships throughout her life, she lived her life with grace, faith in God, and in service to others.

My mother raised me alone after getting divorced from my father when I was three years old. She had a rough go of it from beginning to end and she was so much stronger than she thought. Born in Ireland, she had two sisters and two brothers. Tragically, her mother contracted tuberculosis and died at the age of 32. My mother was only three years old. After the age of seven, she never saw her father again because the church came between them. The children had been raised as Protestants and long story short, the church took the children because her father remarried a Catholic woman. His new wife was so generous of spirit that she was willing to take in all the children despite already having three children of her own and having a small two-bedroom home. The church said, "We'll look after them," and they ended up being separated, all in different homes.

At the age of 17, Mom immigrated to the United States on a large ship with her sister Ann and her Aunt Ann. They had to leave her sister Reenie behind because she had a lazy eye. In those days, immigrants were rejected if found to have health defects, even one as minor as a lazy eye. It was tragic because Reenie ended up in an abusive marriage and she died at a young age. At least now, they are reunited in heaven.

My mother served in the Army and the Air Force in the late 1950s. She was married twice and divorced twice and sadly never found love again. She dedicated her life to raising me and my two brothers. She worked nights so she could be there for us during the day. This took a toll on her body. She also suffered from depression, and she was injured in several car accidents. She faced a lot of health problems as she got older, and I just wanted to help her.

She is the reason I started to investigate alternative medicine. She used to say that I kept her alive. I was no match against the pandemic though. I couldn't help her. I never felt so helpless and distraught. Before that, I was always able to go to her and be with her and support her, cook for her, bring her healthy teas, supplements, and foods, as well as lots of cheer.

She joined me in learning and researching. She would read to me over the phone about remedies. She would call me with questions about things to research on the internet. So, I would look up whatever she wanted. Anytime she was prescribed a new medication, I would read about it to her over the phone. One day, I examined her lab work and found that she had elevated ANA antibodies, which indicated she had autoimmune disease. I asked her doctor to run a thyroid panel. It turned out that she had elevated TSH and elevated TPO antibodies. Her diagnosis had been MISSED for decades, thus contributing to the development of many additional health problems. Her doctors had never treated her thyroid autoimmune illness. All they did was send her to a rheumatologist. I remember her telling me that the rheumatologist did nothing for her. She suffered unnecessarily for years. She trusted them. She was a victim of our profit-based healthcare system. At one point, she had vertigo and was holding on to furniture and walls just to walk through her apartment. I reviewed her medications and discovered her doctor had her on 18 medications! I wrote him a three-page letter detailing her history, her symptoms, and my concern about the excessive number of medications. I made a connection between the medications and the side effects she was experiencing. Soon after that, he removed 10 medications, which resulted in her taking only eight medications daily. The vertigo was resolved. He had been adding more and more medication, without regard for the interactions and repercussions. You must advocate for your family members, especially seniors.

So, Mom . . . this book is dedicated to you. I know you are always with us. I love when you visit me in my dreams and send birds my way. I love you so much.

This book is also dedicated to all the exhausted, long-suffering moms out there who receive inadequate care from their doctors and are continuously searching for answers on how to feel better. I hope you find some answers here.

Medical Disclaimer

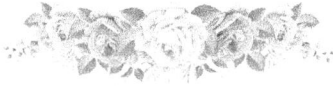

As a reader of this material, you understand this book is for informational purposes only and does not provide health care, medical, or nutrition therapy services. It does not diagnose, treat, or cure any disease, condition, or other physical or mental ailment of the human body. It is not to be used as a replacement or substitute for medical advice provided by physicians and trained medical professionals. If you are under the care of a healthcare professional or are currently using prescription medications, you should discuss any dietary changes, dietary supplements, exercise programs, and any other changes with your physician, and should not discontinue any prescription medications without first consulting your doctor.

Contents

Introduction

This is not your usual thyroid book. I have lived it. I have been very physically ill, and I've also suffered the depression and anxiety that often accompany thyroid disease. I've been depleted of my strength and vitality after numerous injuries, losses, and traumas. I developed thyroid nodules after going undiagnosed for years, and I feared cancer, but I picked myself up and I learned. I experimented with superfoods, herbal elixirs, and megadoses of specific nutrients. I detoxed my body in several ways on multiple occasions and treated myself with many types of holistic medicine. I shrunk my thyroid nodules and I have restored all my thyroid lab numbers to normal levels. I only take one medication which is mostly overlooked by doctors but helps so many people with autoimmune disease and other conditions.

I am not a doctor, which means I can speak freely about effective and scientifically proven natural medicine. I will tell you the truth about how holistic treatment is safer and more effective than traditional medical treatment for Hashimoto's, hypothyroidism, and detoxification treatment. If my message is successful, I will save many thyroid glands and help many people, mostly women, to recover their health safely.

I'm writing this book to teach people with Hashimoto's disease how to:

- Reclaim your health and feel happy and energetic again
- Become empowered to heal yourself with safe and effective holistic medicine
- Avoid the need for thyroid removal surgery and repeated biopsies
- Detox heavy metals or other toxins without recirculating the toxins and feeling horrible
- Discover and treat hidden infections
- Prevent your condition from worsening and progressing to other autoimmune diseases or cancer

I share many wonderful health-promoting gems with you that you will not hear from your doctors. I tend to find information that most people have never heard about. How do I know that? Usually because when I am connecting with an individual, they either ask me questions, or have an expression of surprise, delight, or confusion. I love seeing the look on their face when I share HOPE with them. When I share a CURE with them. When I get them EXCITED to jump in and take the next step to get WELL.

Most importantly, I'm writing this book with the hope that I can show people that it can be done, thus empowering them. Knowledge is power and your mindset is a huge force in your healing process. Believing you can heal motivates you to take the steps to make it happen. I want to save people from suffering and wasting time searching for answers. I want to help people believe that it can be done because it HAS been done. You can do it too!

I have 30 years of experience as a technical writer and it's an important goal for me to publish a book and to use my writing skills for a higher purpose. I didn't set out to be a writer, but I moved into technical writing after being a software developer for several years.

I graduated with degrees in Computer Science and Psychology in my twenties and have studied alternative healing in my spare time ever since. As I researched how to help Mom with her health problems, I discovered that natural health and nutrition was my passion. There's an endless world of possibilities. I studied herbology, nutrition, Ayurveda, Chinese medicine, Native American herbs, South American herbs, superfoods, essential oils, and many healing modalities. I learned about flower essences, light therapy, colon therapy, frequency healing, meditation, spiritual healing, ear candling, and more. I feel a strong spiritual faith and I know that I have a mission to help people, whether it's just by giving them a smile, a laugh, a health tip, or whatever I am guided to do. If someone is ill, I'm driven to help them but I have learned not to push if people are not ready or willing to accept the information.

I studied at the Institute for Integrative Nutrition (IIN) and graduated in December 2012 as a Certified Integrative Health Coach. I then became a board-certified drugless practitioner with the American Association of Drugless Practitioners (AADP). I also studied with the Clayton College of Natural Health, and I've taken many classes, and attended many events, webinars, and health summits.

I cannot tell you how incredible the experience at IIN was. I was taught by some of the most amazing teachers. We studied over 110 diets. We learned how to coach people not only with information but with heart and compassion. The teachers at IIN were perfectly selected, and they were truly wonderful communicators. I still follow many of them and continue to learn from them.

Part of the reason I appreciate and cherish my year at IIN is because it was the year that I felt the absolute worst physically. My energy was on the floor. My adrenals were shot. I had sprained my ankle and herniated four disks in my neck. I was struggling as a single mother raising two boys, one with autism and severe ADHD, and one with ADHD. Some people don't like to label, but we are all officially diagnosed, and we live it, and it's the easiest way to convey the situation for the purposes of this book. I treat my children like normal wonderful people, which they ARE.

There were behavioral challenges, especially at school, for my youngest with autism. There were many times I had to leave work for my children. I was commuting 45 minutes back and forth to work, and I was struggling with a very heavy workload. I started to fall apart. I was depressed and anxious, but I tried not to show it. The happiest part of my day was picking up my kids, and then picking up my iPad and attending IIN classes where I found great inspiration. The lectures elevated my mood and my energy. I had found my tribe.

The following year, I was accepted to write as a Citizen Journalist for *Natural News*. I published several articles, including one in December 2013, titled, "Woman Shrinks Thyroid Nodules with Natural Medicine".[1] This article provides a brief description of how I shrunk my thyroid nodules. In this book, I go into far more detail about how I went into remission, shrunk my thyroid nodules, and how I continue to improve and maintain my health.

In 2016, I studied a different nutrition program and earned the David Wolfe Nutrition certification from the Body Mind Institute (now known as UEXL Institute). In 2017, my study focused on essential oils, and I earned a Certification in Aromatherapy.

I continue to learn, investigate, and practice to find remedies and treatments to help others to heal. So many people are ill, especially now that there are so many chemicals and contaminants in our food and environment. There are safe and effective ways to heal, and I love to share that information with others.

I feel significantly better now at 55 than I did 11 years ago. I have more energy. I usually feel happy and calm, even though I have been through so much. Getting my body, mind, and spirit in balance has given me a firmer foundation which helps me to handle what life throws at me with more resilience.

So far, I have healed myself naturally from Hashimoto's disease, thyroid nodules, eczema, cystic acne and boils, bronchitis, herniated disks and sprained ankles, ovarian and fibroid cysts, parasites, candida, chronic fatigue, constipation, heavy metal poisoning, and various allergies. I understand how it feels to be faced with serious health problems. My mission is to teach and empower others to heal using natural, safe, and effective methods. I have spent thousands of dollars and countless hours researching and experimenting with various types of alternative healing modalities and using natural medicine in effective combinations that allowed me to heal.

After decades of researching natural healing, I have built a huge library of information, a solid network of experts to gather information from, and a deep knowledge base that helps me to evaluate new information and weed out ineffective products or treatments that don't serve me. I have conquered my fears and I strive to live in a state of love. I feel confident that I can heal whatever I face. I think positively and I try new things with an open mind.

This book details my journey and explains how I was able to shrink my thyroid nodules and conquer Hashimoto's by normalizing my thyroid lab numbers, while also resolving fatigue, depression, anxiety, hair and skin problems, weight gain, and more.

This book teaches you about how to identify and address root causes, detoxification issues, and nutrient deficiencies. You will learn about all the types of thyroid nodules, what the risks of thyroid surgery include, and many ways to prevent cancer and avoid surgery.

This book also includes a thyroid nodule reduction program as well as a comprehensive guide to healing that focuses on mind, body, and spirit. You will learn about iodine, gut healing, nutraceuticals, immune modulators, antiviral herbs, essential oils, and much more.

I will show you how to conquer Hashimoto's autoimmune disease and many of the symptoms that result from this condition.

As you address your root causes and progress through this healing journey, you too will regain your energy, health, and happiness.

CHAPTER 1

Hashimoto's and Hypothyroidism Defined

"Impossible is not a fact . . . it's an opinion. What's impossible only remains so until someone finds a way to do what others are sure can't be done."
– Tony Robbins

An estimated 50 million people in the United States have autoimmune disorders that cause the immune system to attack healthy cells and tissue.[2] Over 100 different autoimmune diseases have been identified. Hashimoto's disease, also known as Hashimoto's thyroiditis, is the most prevalent of all autoimmune diseases. We need more awareness and better treatment for the people (mostly women) that suffer from this challenging disease.

What is Hashimoto's Disease?

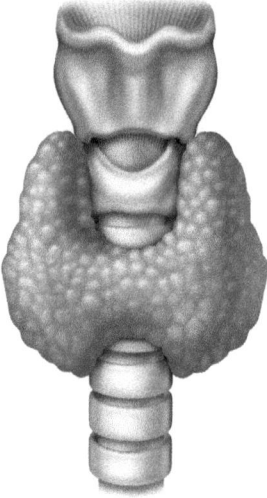

The thyroid gland is an endocrine gland located in the lower front part of the neck below the Adam's apple. It produces hormones that play a role in a variety of functions throughout the body. Thyroid hormones influence weight, growth and development, heart rate, body temperature, and menstrual cycles.

Hashimoto's disease causes immune system cells to attack the thyroid gland. This autoimmune attack creates inflammation in the thyroid tissue, resulting in Hashimoto's thyroiditis. Thyroiditis leads to hypothyroidism which reduces the body's ability to produce hormones. Hashimoto's disease is the most common cause of hypothyroidism.

Approximately **90 percent** of hypothyroidism cases in the United States are caused by Hashimoto's disease.[3] Did you know that? Many people do not due to a lack of knowledge and awareness. Most people with hypothyroidism have an autoimmune disorder and many of them go undiagnosed for years.

While Hashimoto's affects mostly middle-aged women, it also affects men and women of any age, including children. Hashimoto's usually comes on gradually in mid-adulthood, but it sometimes starts earlier or later in life. Childhood traumatic stress was found to increase the likelihood of being diagnosed with autoimmune disease in adulthood.[4] People with Hashimoto's disease have a higher risk of developing other autoimmune disorders, such as vitiligo, lupus, rheumatoid arthritis, type 1 diabetes, Graves' disease, and Addison's disease.

Thyroid Disease Facts

Thyroid disease has skyrocketed over the past few decades. Currently, the American Thyroid Association estimates that approximately 20 million Americans have thyroid disease.[5] Here are some additional facts from the association:

- **Hypo**thyroidism is a condition where the thyroid gland does not produce enough thyroid hormone. It can cause extreme fatigue, depression, forgetfulness, and weight gain.
- **Hyper**thyroidism is a condition where the thyroid gland produces too much thyroid hormone. It can cause weight loss, heart palpitations, tremors, heat intolerance, and can eventually lead to osteoporosis.
- More than **60 percent** of people with thyroid disease are unaware of their condition and go undiagnosed for years, which allows the disease to progress untreated.
- The thyroid gland is a small gland, but it produces a hormone that affects every cell, tissue, and organ in the body. When you have too little or too much thyroid hormone, it can cause a wide variety of symptoms.
- One in eight women will experience a thyroid problem.
- Women are seven times more likely to develop Hashimoto's thyroiditis than men.
- Most thyroid cancers respond to treatment but a small amount of them can be aggressive. With this book, you will learn about how to prevent cancer.
- Undiagnosed thyroid disease can increase the risk of serious conditions such as cardiovascular disease, infertility, diabetes, and osteoporosis.

- Pregnant women with undiagnosed or poorly treated hypothyroidism have a higher risk of miscarriage, premature birth, and developmental problems in their children.

Thyroid Hormones T3 and T4

The thyroid gland secretes triiodothyronine (T3) and thyroxine (T4). The thyroid produces only 20 percent of T3, the active hormone. The remaining 80 percent comes from T4 that is converted to T3, mainly by the liver.

T3 affects almost every physiological process in the body, including growth and development, body temperature, metabolism, and heart rate. A dysfunctional thyroid creates a hormonal imbalance in the body that disrupts normal metabolic processes such as digestion, body temperature, and energy regulation.

Essentially, the thyroid gland, by producing and regulating T4 and T3, ensures that your body remains in a balanced state of growth, metabolism, and energy utilization.

Hypothyroidism Symptoms

Hypothyroidism occurs when the thyroid gland is underactive and does not produce enough thyroid hormone. It slows many processes in your body and causes a variety of symptoms. How many of these symptoms apply to you? I've experienced all but two of them.

Symptoms of Both Hypothyroidism and Hashimoto's Disease		
Chronic fatigue	Brain fog and memory loss	Stiff and painful joints
Low motivation	Lack of concentration	Weight gain
Puffy face and/or eyes	Exercise intolerance	Insulin resistance
Loss of a third of the outer eyebrow	Muscle pain, weakness, tenderness, and stiffness	Inability to lose weight, even with low calorie dieting and exercise
Hair loss and thinning	Constipation	High cholesterol
Dry skin	Chills or sweating	Hoarse voice
Brittle nails	Heavy or irregular menstrual periods or fertility problems	Enlarged thyroid

Autoimmune or Thyroid Disease?

This is what endocrinologists seem to be missing. Why is this so misunderstood? Is it purposely ignored?

Approximately 90 percent of hypothyroidism is caused by Hashimoto's autoimmune disease.

If you have hypothyroidism and you either don't know you have Hashimoto's, or you think you don't have Hashimoto's disease, you have about a 10 percent chance of being correct. If that's the case, it is time to ask your doctor to run the TPO and TG antibody tests. Approximately 80-90 percent of people with Hashimoto's have elevated TPO antibodies, TG antibodies, or both.[6] If left untreated, your thyroid is attacked by your immune system, thyroid tissue gets destroyed, and that interferes with the production of thyroid hormones. Some people never develop elevated thyroid antibodies but have full-blown Hashimoto's and suffer all the same symptoms. This is referred to as seronegative autoimmune thyroiditis, or serum-negative Hashimoto's.

With seronegative Hashimoto's, the person often has a "hypoechoic pattern" on their thyroid gland, which is revealed by a thyroid ultrasound. A hypoechoic nodule appears darker than the surrounding thyroid tissue. This indicates that those nodules are solid instead of fluid-filled. Although these nodules have a higher chance of becoming cancerous, only about 5 percent of thyroid nodules develop into thyroid cancer. If you have not had a thyroid ultrasound yet, you may want to request a baseline thyroid ultrasound to assess the health of your thyroid gland.

If you have developed a goiter or thyroid nodules, your doctor will recommend a Fine Needle Aspiration (FNA) where cells of your nodules are extracted with a needle to check for cancer cells. If cancer cells are found, your doctor may recommend either a partial or total thyroidectomy (removal of thyroid gland). If you have your thyroid removed, you will need to take thyroid hormone medication for the rest of your life. This can be prevented in many cases, especially if you are in the first three stages of Hashimoto's.

Stages of Hashimoto's Disease

Five stages of Hashimoto's have been identified.

Stage 1: The genetic predisposition exists to develop Hashimoto's, but the person does not have thyroid disease or autoimmune disease. Thyroid function is normal and there is no attack on the thyroid.

Stage 2: Silent autoimmunity. The immune system sees the thyroid gland as a foreign invader. The person has symptoms but their TSH, T3, and T4 are in normal range. Thyroid antibody tests might show elevated thyroid antibodies.

Stage 3: The thyroid loses its ability to produce thyroid hormone properly. At this stage, TSH may be mildly elevated, but T3 and T4 levels are in normal range. This is often referred to as "Subclinical hypothyroidism."

Stage 4: The thyroid gland is failing and cannot produce thyroid hormones. TSH is elevated, and T3 and T4 levels are low. At this point diagnosis is late, but more obvious.

Stage 5: Thyroid gland failure. Additional autoimmune diseases become a problem, such as Rheumatoid Arthritis, Sjogren's, Lupus, Raynaud's, and others. This is why some doctors test annually for additional autoimmune disorders.

At stage five, some doctors test for additional autoimmune disorders but testing for more diseases while doing nothing to prevent it from happening is not a good practice. Prevention is far superior. Follow the keys in this book so you never reach the later stages. However, if you *are* experiencing the later stages, keep reading because it may be possible to regenerate your thyroid gland.

Regenerating the Thyroid Gland

The human body has amazing recuperative abilities. You can still improve your health. Thyroid cells have been known to regenerate. In fact, about 330 billion cells are replaced every day. That is about 1 percent of all cells in the human body. At this rate, 30 trillion cells are replenished in 80 to 100 days—which is the equivalent of a new you!

In fact, an exciting development was recently announced. Stem cell treatment has the **potential to regenerate a thyroid gland** that has been damaged or even surgically removed! The Sernova Cell Pouch Therapy is currently in clinical trials for regenerating thyroid tissues after a thyroidectomy. It is also being studied to treat other diseases including autoimmune disease and diabetes.[7]

Causes of Hashimoto's Disease

Research has shown that there are three issues that must exist for an autoimmune disease to develop or be sustained.

- Environmental (chemical) triggers
- Genetic predisposition
- Intestinal permeability

Chemical Link

A growing body of research indicates that exposure to environmental toxins is a key piece of the thyroid disease puzzle. Our world is more toxic than ever.

Over the past few decades, there has been an increasing number of cases of allergies, autoimmune disease, thyroid disease, and cancer. Since 1940, over 80,000 new chemicals were introduced into our society, our environment, our food, water, and air.[8] How many of these 80,000 chemicals were tested for safety? The EPA has ordered testing for less than 300 of these chemicals.[9]

Is there a link? Of course. We are exposed to toxic pollutants, chemicals, and heavy metals on a regular basis. The thyroid gland is especially vulnerable to many of these toxins, especially those that inhibit iodine uptake, and some of us have gene mutations that make it harder for our bodies to detoxify and eliminate toxins.

Many people just throw up their hands and say what can we do? There is a lot we can do! I'm going to show you how to lower your chemical load and detox safely. Don't throw those hands up. You can't give up, because you could end up feeling worse and developing more health problems, possibly additional autoimmune diseases. You'll learn more about toxins that affect the thyroid, how to avoid them, and how to detox them, in Chapter 6 and Chapter 8.

Genetic Link

You could say that autoimmunity runs in the family, but it's not a foregone conclusion. There is a genetic component but there is not one specific gene that has been shown to cause Hashimoto's. There are several genes however that can make you more susceptible to developing Hashimoto's. Having these genes does not mean you will definitely get Hashimoto's disease. There are a variety of combinations of these genes, and they can be expressed differently in different individuals. New research continues to study genes that affect susceptibility to Hashimoto's.

While genetics play a role in the development of Hashimoto's, it is not a clear relationship. Look at twins. Identical twins share the exact same DNA. If a condition is completely genetic, and one twin has a condition, then the other twin will have the exact same condition 100 percent of the time. However, in studies of twins where one twin is diagnosed with Hashimoto's, the other twin has only a 55 percent chance of developing it. Based on observations made during the clinical practice of Dr. Izabella Wentz, genetic predisposition is only about 25 percent of the risk for developing Hashimoto's, which means you have the ability to change about 75 percent of your risk for Hashimoto's.[10]

We discuss genes and their relationship to health in more detail in Chapter 15.

Intestinal Permeability

Many factors contribute to intestinal problems. One in particular is the heavy use of pesticides and herbicides. Genetically modified foods are heavily sprayed with herbicide that contains glyphosate, a known carcinogen that causes **damage to the gut**. Poor gut health is linked to autoimmune disease, food allergies, and more. See Chapter 10 to learn more about GMO foods and how to heal your gut.

The incidence of autoimmune disease has skyrocketed since the late 1990s. Genetically modified organisms (GMOs) were introduced into our food supply in the 1990s. Coincidence? I don't think so. The only factor? No of course not. But are GMO foods considered by mainstream medicine to be a contributing factor to this epidemic? The Centers for Disease Control and Prevention (CDC) reportedly does not know why rates of autoimmune disease are skyrocketing.

Consider this. Did children have food allergies before the 90s? Allergies in children were practically nonexistent when I was growing up in the 70s and 80s. Hay fever, maybe, but foods, no. We all ate peanut butter and jelly sandwiches for example. We all ate plenty of gluten and dairy. Now it's quite common for children to have allergies.

Research has shown that the increasing use of glyphosate is linked to the growing problem worldwide of gluten intolerance and celiac disease. Even fish exposed to glyphosate developed digestive problems similar to celiac disease.[11] Glyphosate is linked to many diseases and illnesses, including cancer, liver disease, thyroid disease, autism, intestinal permeability, and nutritional deficiencies.[12]

We will dive deeper into the causes of Hashimoto's in Chapter 5 and Chapter 6.

My Diagnosis

Doctors typically diagnose hypothyroidism when they observe a high level of thyroid stimulating hormone (TSH) on a blood test. They then prescribe thyroid hormone medication.

This approach falls short. It's too little, too late. At this point, the disease has progressed, and the doctor is catching the problem after stage three of Hashimoto's.

My TSH has NEVER been elevated on a lab test—not once. If I had followed the current medical model, my TSH may very well be elevated by now. I knew for over 10 years that I had a thyroid problem based on my symptoms, but I was never diagnosed properly because my TSH level was normal. I began to address the issue naturally with diet and supplementation (including selenium) long before I was diagnosed.

I was not diagnosed until about a decade after I had been asking various doctors to test me for thyroid problems. I kept insisting that it was my thyroid. Ultimately a primary care physician referred me to an endocrinologist who finally tested me for thyroid antibodies. My primary doctor could have run the test. I don't understand why she didn't. I now get my antibody levels checked by my primary doctor. The endocrinologist I visited was useless to me other than the antibody test. She wasn't even competent enough to provide my diagnosis to me. I saw her writing on her pad, "consistent with Hashimoto's." She wasn't even going to tell me! Thank God I was able to read her writing from across the room. I had wasted enough time going from doctor to doctor. I was obviously an astute patient that was looking for answers.

I tried to engage her in discussion about certain foods and other issues such as iodine, and she had ZERO to say. She just looked at me with a placating smile. When I asked her if she wrote "Hashimoto's," she admitted that it was my diagnosis. She then prescribed levothyroxine, told me to come back in six months, and rushed out of the room. I was puzzled at the time about why she withheld my diagnosis. Later, after looking back and thinking about how I struggled for so many years to get answers, I became frustrated. I was deeply disappointed. I didn't have any more time to waste. I knew I could address my health issues if I just knew what I was dealing with. I had already been healing myself with holistic medicine for several years.

I knew a lot about thyroid medications already. I had researched them. I didn't fill the levothyroxine prescription. I did not want a synthetic form of thyroid hormone. She simply followed the mainstream protocol, which I call the "cookie-cutter" approach.

Do thyroid medications stop the immune system from attacking the thyroid? No, but they are helpful for those with low thyroid hormone levels. The good news is that it is possible to correct your health so that your body starts producing thyroid hormone on its own. See Chapter 6 for more information about thyroid hormones and testing.

Destructive Effects of Dodgy Diagnosis

The "standard of care" for most endocrinologists and primary care doctors is to look at TSH (thyroid stimulating hormone) and T4 levels to screen for hypothyroidism. These two tests do not provide an accurate diagnosis. People are suffering (as I did) with hypothyroidism symptoms for years before receiving any kind of diagnosis. People often suffer with thyroid symptoms for 10 years or more before receiving treatment or diagnosis. Many are offered antidepressant medications and even birth control pills to treat their symptoms.

As the disease progresses and ultimately starts to impact the TSH and T4 levels, physicians start to treat the thyroid with thyroid hormone medication without addressing the autoimmune disease and what is causing it. They don't differentiate between non-autoimmune thyroid issues and Hashimoto's autoimmune disease. They often miss the subtle fluctuations of thyroid hormones and elevated thyroid antibodies that occur in the early stages of Hashimoto's and hypothyroidism. Why do they lag so far behind? If it was a more serious disease, those patients might not survive for 10 years. The "standard of care" is not *care* in my opinion. It's neglect. It neglects the root causes of the illness and neglects the symptoms of the patient.

Functional Medicine Dives Deeper

Functional medicine doctors take more time to evaluate the patient. They utilize specialized training and techniques to identify the root causes of complex illnesses. They spend time discussing symptoms, lifestyle, diet, medications, supplements, and more, to get a full picture of what is going on with the patient. They work with patients to resolve the root causes of their illness which can resolve the issue or prevent worsening of the condition.

With patients that exhibit symptoms of hypothyroidism, they review the full thyroid lab panel to evaluate if a patient has "cellular hypothyroidism." On the surface, it may appear that all the numbers on lab work are normal because they are within the specified ranges, but with functional medicine, doctors look at numbers that are on the lower or upper end of the ranges. They evaluate the ratios of T3 to Reverse T3, and Free T3 to Reverse T3. They also evaluate metabolism, inflammation, adrenal function, allergies, toxicities, and more.

According to WebMD, functional medicine doctors "may be ideal for people with chronic illnesses that aren't easily managed by conventional medical techniques."[13] If that is the case and they know this, then mainstream doctors should refer patients to functional medicine doctors instead of leaving them to flounder and search for answers on their own. In my opinion, **functional medicine should be fully covered by health insurance plans**. I think that would significantly lower healthcare costs by preventing and reversing a lot of illnesses.

Imagine the amount of suffering, time, and money that could be saved by preventing the onset of serious disease by making functional and preventative medicine an integrated part of our medical system. By employing a multi-faceted approach to autoimmunity, focusing on diet, detox, and gut healing, we can set the stage for our bodies to heal from autoimmunity. And with time, we can completely reverse most (or all) of our worst symptoms. You will learn in the coming chapters how to find and resolve issues that can lead to autoimmunity and other health issues.

CHAPTER 2

The Stormy Road to Sickness

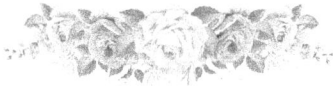

"My mission in life is not merely to survive, but to thrive; and to do so with some passion, some compassion, some humor, and some style."
— Maya Angelou

Many elements factored into my body turning autoimmune. If I only knew then what I know now! Living with illness is not easy, but I am determined to stay positive and keep working on it, having faith that everything will be okay. When I am feeling great, I try to figure out what I am doing right. When I am not feeling well, I evaluate what am doing wrong. I am on a quest for better health, not just for myself, but so I can help others.

Healing Hashimoto's has been a journey of highs and lows. I went from feeling weak, fatigued, heavy, and depressed to feeling happy and energetic most of the time. Shrinking my thyroid nodules was probably the most exciting part of this journey, but not the most significant. Staying healthy, cancer free, and living with energy, stamina, and a clear productive mind is the most rewarding accomplishment because these are long-term results that affect my quality of life every day. Inflammation caused by Hashimoto's can lead to a lot of different problems, including pain, stiffness, and blurry vision. Sometimes, I'm too busy to even think about it, but I try to discover the root causes of my symptoms and address them by adjusting my diet and lifestyle choices.

I can say with certainty after being diagnosed in 2012 my condition has significantly improved, and I feel better at 55 than I did at 44 years of age. I've become more productive. I wrote this book after all. It was a labor of love and I feel optimistic that it will help many people. In contrast, in the first few years after becoming ill, I was so fatigued that many other things in my life fell behind. I did the best I could on all fronts. My priority had to be work and my kids. I have a challenging career and commuting was a big drain. At home, things were a mess, and my ex didn't understand. He did fixer-upper projects, but he didn't help in the house. He would just criticize me. He expected me to manage all the cooking, cleaning, shopping, bills, and childcare. He had no idea how hard it was for me just to get the basics done. It was a lot just to make sure the kids were fed, bathed, homework and laundry done, kitchen clean, and garbage taken out. After working all day and taking care of the kids, I had no energy left so weekends were spent doing housework, cooking, and shopping.

After improving my health, I found myself having a second wind in the evenings and now I have continuous energy throughout the day on most days. I even have trouble falling asleep. I enjoy staying up late and getting things done or just relaxing and watching some television.

My energy is higher than it's been in years. I believe that's because my adrenal gland health has improved. You will learn about your adrenal glands and how to support them in Chapter 5 and Chapter 13.

One of the things that many of us struggle with is chronic stress and taking on too much. Sometimes life just doesn't slow down, and self-care doesn't get the highest priority. We should all make ourselves a priority, especially when we are not feeling our best. Stress and illness can lead to adrenal fatigue, and you don't want that.

You might learn some things in this book that you have never heard before. Some may go in one ear and out the other. I urge you to hold on to the key learnings. You may want to bookmark or highlight pages that spark your curiosity and review the information again later. If something sounds incredible, don't presume it's too good to be true.

It's interesting how we need repeated exposure to ideas in general before accepting or acting on them. This is especially true when it comes to our health. I've experienced this myself. I've heard about certain concepts, supplements, remedies, or foods over the years many times before I adopted them into my life.

For example, while studying herbology and natural medicine, alfalfa popped up on more than one occasion. Many of us think of alfalfa as food for cows or other animals or we may never think about it at all. But it's an amazing plant that provides not only vitamins and minerals but is also a source of protein. For people who are vegan or vegetarian, this is a solid source of protein and many other nutrients that can extend your life span by strengthening your blood vessels while normalizing your blood sugar and blood pressure. This helps to prevent cardiovascular disease and helps with respiratory disorders. It also builds the blood. Its seeds or dried leaves can be consumed as a supplement, or the seeds can be sprouted and eaten in the form of alfalfa sprouts. Alfalfa is rich in vitamin K, which is hard to get in foods. It helps in the process of building healthy bones and helps your blood clot so injuries can heal. Vitamin K may even reduce your risk of cardiovascular disease. Besides vitamin K, alfalfa contains vitamin C, folate, thiamine, riboflavin, magnesium, iron, and copper. Many plants are just amazing. You won't see an ad or commercial for them though!

My question to you is: Why wait? Time is of the essence. If I can tell you about effective nutrients that can improve your quality of life, wouldn't you want to know so you can take action right away? I've wasted a lot of time by not acting right away because I either forgot or got sidetracked. However, over the years, I've experimented with many foods, therapies, and supplements. I will share with you what made the biggest difference for me.

I have been using and studying holistic medicine since the early 1990s. The power of natural medicine, superfoods, and super herbs fascinates me and gives me hope. It's my passion. I don't remember exact conversations or the names of all my neighbors, but I remember the cures for many conditions and diseases, and I remember the benefits of all the top super herbs, supplements, essential oils, and foods! I've had many successes and positive experiences with healing various health issues. I love to use that knowledge to help my family and other people to heal and improve their lives.

When I Got Sick

Looking back, I think I started having a thyroid imbalance after my first child was born when I was 30 years old. I was very tired and gained a lot of weight, and I developed eczema. I had to return to work when my baby was only seven weeks old because we had just bought a house and needed my income. My ex-husband had a long commute and would arrive home tired, leaving me with all the household and baby responsibilities. I was under a lot of stress but very happy to be a mother.

Eczema Hell

I developed a horrible case of eczema on my hands after the birth of my first son. Only my ring finger was affected for the most part. I used to joke that I was allergic to being married! I had a jeweler put a platinum coating on the inside. That was a waste of money. It was extremely itchy and irritating. It peeled and oozed. I visited several doctors and none of them were able to help. I was prescribed a steroid cream that resulted in the skin on my fingers cracking. That was painful and very irritating when performing household tasks. The doctor never warned me that the steroid cream was only supposed to be applied for only a few weeks. I continued to apply the cream for several months. After learning that the cracks in my skin were a side effect of the steroid cream, I ceased using it and sought alternatives.

I tried many things to cure my eczema and eventually succeeded but it took almost 10 years. I stopped eating dairy temporarily. That helped somewhat. I had all my amalgam (mercury) fillings removed. I discovered that a drink with sucralose gave me a severe skin reaction and worsened my eczema. I eliminated sucralose and it improved but the eczema remained on my fingers. I took fish oil, borage oil, and evening primrose oil at different times. I tried flaxseed oil and black seed oil, but I could not stomach the taste. For months, I drank a tablespoon of chlorophyll juice daily which gave me a nice green smile. If you ever tried it, you know how rich that green color is! I drank many green drinks and made bone broth. I also used countless colon cleanse products, probiotics, triphala, and collagen products. I eliminated gluten. All these things helped to heal my gut over time.

There are several types of eczema. Some people think it's caused by allergies to detergents, metals, or other elements. However, those types of reactions are more likely to be dermatitis. Eczema is different. It is caused by an internal imbalance. It can be very difficult to cure, but it's possible. First and foremost, you must heal your gut. Also make sure you have a healthy vitamin D level.

The first time I was tested for my vitamin D level, it was 40 (range: 30–100). I was at the lower end of the range. I started taking 10,000 UI daily of vitamin D3 gel caps (with olive oil, not soy). I was able to bring my vitamin D level up above 60 and I felt significantly better. Do not underestimate the importance of your vitamin D level. Some doctors prescribe 50,000 UI or higher to help patients raise their levels quickly. I chose to do it gradually.

I have been completely cured of eczema for about 15 years. I have also resolved a lot of allergies, including allergies to animals, foods, and environmental allergens. This took time. There is no quick fix. It involved taking steps to heal my gut and modulate my immune system.

Straw Hair and Missing Brows

After the birth of my second son, my hair dried up to the point where it was like straw. I would wake up in the morning, and all my hair would be tangled up on my head like a bird's nest. That was embarrassing and alarming. Fortunately, it was temporary.

The outer third of my eyebrows disappeared. This is a common symptom of hypothyroidism. At this point, I knew something was wrong with my thyroid. I am happy to say that my eyebrows grew back and look fine now, and my hair is long and healthy.

Fatigue and Heaviness

My energy hit the floor. It's different than normal tiredness or sleep deprivation. It's like your body is wrung out like a dish rag, depleted, done. Getting up was a huge effort. I felt like I weighed a thousand pounds as I walked up the stairs. I used to pile things up on the steps just so I could make fewer trips up and down. One day I slipped on some of those items and fell hard on my tailbone. I was carrying my son who was two years old at the time, and I braced him for the fall and took the whole brunt of it. I learned what seeing stars meant that day. Poor Adrian was crying, and we were all alone. It took me a while to get up. I just held my baby boy and comforted him.

A few years later, a doctor finally tested my adrenal function and told me my adrenals were shot. When I was with my ex, he didn't understand my fatigue. He would complain and tell me that I take too many breaks. I just didn't have the strength. He didn't understand what I was going through. A lot of spouses don't understand because it's not a disease that is clearly understood. Your symptoms are invisible to others. People see the weight gain but might just assume you are lazy or eat too much. The lack of energy and lack of understanding is frustrating, but it can be solved. I have lots of energy now. It went up in increments. It feels wonderful to have energy again. If you are suffering with fatigue, hang in there. One step at a time. It will come back.

Autism Undiagnosed in my Son

The stories of my boys are not the subject of this book, but I would be remiss not to mention how the birth of my children affected my health. My immune system started to attack my thyroid after the birth of my second child. It was certainly not his fault of course but it is common for many women with Hashimoto's to become ill soon after the birth of a child.

My second baby boy, Adrian, was born with autism. I suspected it right away because he had poor eye contact and he didn't like being held. This was in contrast to my first son, Adam, who was a sweet cuddler and who stared right into my eyes as soon as he was placed into my arms. Adrian was very sensitive to noise and touch, and his speech and toilet training were delayed. Many signs of autism were there, but I had to tell the doctor the diagnosis. Several pediatricians failed to diagnose or test him. I find it interesting when I hear people say, "Our son was diagnosed with autism by our pediatrician." Really? I took my son to several pediatricians and told them that I thought he had autism, but none of them officially diagnosed him or helped in any way. Finally, after visiting a child psychiatrist, he was officially diagnosed and treated.

Adrian had pink patches of eczema on both cheeks as a baby, leading me to think he had gut issues. Gut issues are very common in children with autism. I fed him yogurt and gave him chewable probiotics and after a few months, his face cleared up. Once he started walking and talking, it was non-stop pandemonium. There was mess everywhere, fights with his brother, broken items, and cereal everywhere. It was virtually impossible to keep the house clean. It was challenging to go to certain events such as parades because of the noise. He still hates parades. Certain noises are physically painful to his ears.

Once he went to school, there were behavioral issues all the way from pre-school through middle school. His principal and several of his teachers did not seem to be properly trained in how to deal with autistic children. He went through several years in school where he just was not engaged, and he was punished excessively. He was put in situations that were impossible for a child with his disabilities to deal with, including loud gym events, such as pep rallies. They should have given him noise-canceling headphones, but they didn't. When my son would react, he was often punished. I was called at work many times to come and get him. This was happening as early as second grade. At one point, he went through a phase where he wanted to hug people a lot. I think it helped to soothe him. The school declared a new rule based on Adrian—NO more hugs! Can you imagine? Sure, he may have hugged a little too much, but that was so unkind. Later, it happened again with high fives! No more high fives! Poor boy. He had so much pent-up energy. They also punished him by taking away recess. I suggested extra homework and offered to help him with it, but they stuck to their guns. No recess. No outlet.

Some situations left me so depleted and depressed. Once I was invited to a meeting at the school where I was completely outnumbered. There were 10 people sitting around a table, and one by one, they went around the table trashing my son, voicing their complaints and criticisms, and making me feel terrible. He never did those things at home. I felt saddened and defeated, like a steamroller drove over me. I went home and cried my eyes out and drowned my sorrows. I felt so alone because his father never entered the school to support me for any of his IEP meetings or summons to the principal's office. He would say, "I have to work," and he would never make the time to help. In the meantime, I had a long commute to work, and I had to fulfill my responsibilities as a Lead Technical Writer, while the kids went to aftercare at the end of the school day. Then I would race home to pick them both up on time, and do dinner, homework, baths, etc. It was truly exhausting. My only break was when they went with their fathers on some weekends. Most of my me-time was spent alone doing laundry and housework. The stress was certainly a contributing factor to my autoimmunity in retrospect.

In middle school, Adrian finally had a teacher that he could communicate with, that understood him, and showed him compassion and interest. He started to grow and progress quickly. He flourished with her. She lives close by and sometimes we visit her. We will always love and appreciate Mrs. Jessie Francisco. She turned everything around for Adrian.

I always knew Adrian was highly intelligent. Once he started high school, he matured and figured out how to behave well and earn good grades. He never got in trouble again! In fact, he achieved honor roll several times. I was never summoned to the principal's office. Whenever we saw his high school principal, he greeted us with a smile. What a refreshing change! Now, Adrian socializes well at work and with friends and he is a helpful family member. He is honest and conscientious, and he has developed a very strong character. Now he helps to alleviate my stress, helps me in the house, and makes me laugh every day. My boys are both wonderful sons.

Postpartum Thyroiditis

Approximately 5–10 percent of women experience postpartum thyroiditis (PPT).[14] I didn't know about PPT at the time, but I later learned that many women are diagnosed with Hashimoto's after the birth of a child. After my second son was born, I noticed my hair turned to straw. That had never happened before. The outer third of my eyebrows fell out. I gained weight. I had trouble concentrating and dreaded going back to work. I was in love with my baby boy, and my entire focus was on him and my eldest son. I visited a doctor to discuss my symptoms and I suggested that I had a thyroid problem. My TSH was normal, so my concern was dismissed. I wish my doctor would have told me about PPT.

PPT can be a temporary condition and can be treated with thyroid hormone or if it's mild, it can go untreated. After six to 12 months of thyroid hormone therapy, medication is stopped to determine if long-term or permanent treatment is needed. According to the American Thyroid Organization, most women regain normal thyroid function within 12 to 18 months after the onset of symptoms. However, approximately 20 percent of those that go into a hypothyroid phase will remain hypothyroid.

How to Prevent PPT

A study published in the *Journal of Clinical Endocrinology & Metabolism* found that pregnant women with elevated Thyroid Peroxidase Antibodies (TPOAb) are prone to develop PPT and permanent hypothyroidism. In this study, one group of mothers received 200 mcg of selenium daily and the other group received a placebo. The results showed that selenium supplementation during pregnancy and in the postpartum period reduced thyroid inflammation and the incidence of hypothyroidism.[15]

Imagine if OB/GYNs in all selenium-deficient regions of the world advised pregnant mothers to supplement with selenium. If only this was done, perhaps a lot of needless suffering could be prevented, leaving mothers to focus on mothering.

Annual Bronchitis

I used to suffer occasionally with bronchitis as a girl. My mother told me I inherited it from my father. I also suffered from bronchitis many times throughout my twenties and thirties.

It could be a genetic weakness but it's certainly not unsurmountable. I have not had bronchitis for about 15 years now. I have done a lot of things to improve my immunity, but I think that increasing my vitamin D level was the main factor in preventing reoccurrences of bronchitis. After taking 10,000 UI daily of vitamin D3 for a year, my level was above 60. This made a huge improvement in my health. I never suffered bronchitis again. Not once! No more hacking for a month every time I got sick with a cold. I used to cough so much that I would strain my chest and back muscles and I would be in pain all over my upper body.

Severe Stress

Stressful events can take a toll on your health. We all know that. However, severe stressors often coincide with the onset of autoimmune disease. For example, losing a loved one, going through a divorce, or losing a job.

There were several highly stressful events that preceded my autoimmune diagnosis.

Divorce

Going through a divorce is a deep and painful loss. In 2001, my ex-husband and I started the divorce process. It was amicable, but still very painful. I was very lonely and depressed. About a year after we split up, I met my ex-fiancé. We fell in love and had a son but did not get married. I think I knew it was best not to, because I didn't think it would last and it didn't. We split up after six years. I was 40 years old. Again, I felt like I had lost my family, and I was emotionally distraught for a long time. I did a lot of spiritual therapy and soul-searching. I spent a lot of time alone, grieving, healing, reading, praying, and regaining my strength.

Losing my Father

My father's health started to fail after he turned 60. He had a heart attack, suffered a serious fall, and later had several mini strokes. He lost his ability to walk normally. I managed his care in a couple of nursing homes ultimately moving him to New Jersey where I could visit more often. Simultaneously, I managed his seven-unit apartment building which was a four-hour drive away. My dad passed away on December 11, 2010. He was 67 years old. After he passed, I noticed a lot of butterflies around me, even when I was driving down the highway, which was unusual. I knew he was sending them.

Landlady Hell

Dad's property was close to my mom's home so I would pack up the kids and lots of goodies for mom and make the drive every few months. It was draining. Some tenants are good, and some are very destructive. I'll never be a landlady again. Dealing with tenants in Sterling, CT was often a nightmare. There were no police in that town. People initially would say anything to get in, and then they would either stop paying rent, or become hateful and destructive.

Some of them were filthy. One man did not own a mop and never cleaned his floors, then complained about having mice. Filth attracts rodents! He would trap them and release them outside so they could run right back in. One crazy lady was a realtor and I thought she would be a good tenant. Instead, she never paid a dollar of rent, and when I told her to move out, she nailed the windows shut and changed the door lock so we couldn't get in.

Many of them abused drugs. People were seen running up the hill through the woods to buy drugs from a crazy young couple that had fist fights in the parking lot and left a massive hole in the wall inside their apartment. Property was damaged countless times. Apartments were destroyed and rehabbed multiple times. Eventually, the septic system failed, and I paid to connect the sewage system to the city sewer. I also had to pay to rebuild a three-story outdoor staircase, and much of the roof. I didn't make a dime of profit over the whole seven years. I was lucky to breakeven. What a waste. So much stress—for nothing! I wish I had sold the property years earlier.

Extreme Workload

While managing tenants and raising two children, I was under enormous pressure, and was not feeling very well. I asked my manager at the time if I could work at home after spraining my ankle and being diagnosed with four herniated disks in my neck. She initially agreed, but virtually doubled my workload. I was working at home but putting in 60 to 70 hours of work per week. My project manager said I was doing more work than anyone else on the team. I was exhausted and reached my lowest point. I felt like my heart was slowing down. It was difficult going up and down the stairs. My health was declining. When I finally spoke up and complained about the workload, my manager reversed her decision and demanded I commute to the office. I was driving with an ice pack on my neck barely able to move my neck, which was dangerous. When I confided in an official at the company, they recognized that she did not honor an accommodation letter from my doctor, and they offered me a severance package. With that, I decided to resign and take some time to recover. I took about six months off work and completed my health coaching program.

Mom's Chronic Illness and Death

All this time, my mother had been suffering with chronic illness. Whenever I went to the rental property in Connecticut, I stayed with my mom, brought her health supplements, gifts, food, and treats, and spent time with her. My mom was a gentle and kind Christian woman, originally from the beautiful emerald isle, Ireland. She was witty, intelligent, and kind. She loved me and my two brothers unconditionally. She and I traveled often together. We went to California, Florida, Delaware, Montreal, New York, Maine, Massachusetts, and Puerto Rico. We visited Ireland together twice in the 90s. I will always cherish those memories.

Tragically, my mom passed away from Covid-19 on April 23, 2020, at age 84. It was the most painful experience of my life. It could have been prevented but New Jersey Governor Murphy mandated specific rules restricting use of masks and gowns in the veteran's nursing homes early in the pandemic which contributed to the spread. In addition, Covid-19-positive people were moved in with other patients, and that's exactly what they did to my mother. A couple days after the sick woman was moved into her room, the fever began, and they moved her to the Covid ward. I couldn't call her anymore. A lot of awful things happened, and it was heart-wrenching for me because I couldn't be there by her side. It was also hard to get the doctors and nurses on the phone.

She had been doing better until the pandemic started. She moved into the veteran's nursing home in New Jersey on January 10, 2020. She had suffered multiple falls at her home and she needed a lot of care after breaking her humerus bone. Having her close by was such a relief at first because I was able to get her better care with my doctors, and I was able to go visit every day or two, and eat with her, and bring her surprises. She and I had plans to do many things together, including going shopping and visiting the Jersey shore. But then suddenly, I was shut out. From March 11, 2020, I was no longer allowed to go in and visit her.

This is a very sad time that I don't wish to describe in detail in this book but my wonderful mom is an important part of my story. Let me just say that I love and miss her very much. I brought her to New Jersey so I could be there for her every day and hold her hand until the end, but instead she had to die alone and that still devastates me. I don't know if I'll ever get over it. She deserved so much better. She needed me and she deserved to have me there at her side at the end of her life.

CHAPTER 3

Shrinking Thyroid Nodules

"Imagine a world in which medicine was oriented toward healing rather than disease, where doctors believed in the natural healing capacity of human beings and emphasized prevention above treatment. In such a world, doctors and patients would be partners working toward the same ends."
– Dr. Andrew Weil

In 2013, I visited a doctor who was recommended to me by a coworker. He was an elderly fellow, and I was hopeful his experience would be beneficial. As I was telling him about my symptoms, he leaned his head back and closed his eyes. I was telling him how I felt depressed, fatigued, and I was breaking out, etc. With his eyes closed he chanted quietly, "Prozaaaaaac . . .

birth controooool . . ." I was sitting across from him observing him in his trance-like state just saying the names of medications. I found it strange and funny and did not plan to take any of those medications! First off, I knew the side effects of the meds he rattled off. Secondly, I knew that even if they helped, they were only band aids to treat the symptoms, and would not cure me because they had nothing to do with my root causes. I call him Dr. TrancePharm.

First Thyroid Ultrasound

Dr. TrancePharm did do something helpful though. When he saw that my Thyroid Peroxidase antibodies (TPO) were high, he asked me if I would like an ultrasound of my thyroid, and I agreed. I was very curious to see how my thyroid looked. I had been experiencing thyroid disease symptoms for about 10 years at that point. It was the first ultrasound I had ever received of my thyroid, and it came back with disturbing results. It revealed that I had two thyroid nodules. The larger one was 1.3 cm. The smaller one was 0.9 mm.

He referred me to an endocrinologist, who I call Dr. CuttThroat. You'll see why. He reviewed my ultrasound and said I had two nodules, and one was considered large at 1.3 cm. A thyroid nodule is a growth of thyroid cells that gravitate into a lump within one of the lobes of the thyroid. They can be either solid or filled with fluid (cystic). Most thyroid nodules are benign. However, the doctor created further worry on my part by stating that it was solid and had uneven edges, which meant the risk for cancer was higher. Instead of a 5–10 percent risk of cancer, it was 10–15 percent. The odds were in my favor, but I was still worried.

I asked him what would happen if it was cancer. He did not respond verbally. He literally motioned with his hand, making a **cut your throat hand-motion** across his own neck. Well, that gesture was not only unprofessional, but it was also insensitive, unethical, and just plain disgusting. I was worried about having cancer. It was nothing to joke about. Thus, the name Dr. CuttThroat. I truly hope he didn't do that to anyone else. In any case, he didn't get to slice **my** throat!

Thyroid Needle Biopsy

Dr. CuttThroat referred me to get a needle biopsy which is called a fine needle aspiration (FNA). I asked him if I could wait a little while before getting the biopsy so that I could try some natural medicine. He asked how long, and I suggested two months. He agreed, so I went ahead with my program. I would have done it whether he agreed or not because I believe in the power of holistic medicine and the situation was not dire.

I have a great deal of respect for doctors, and I always listen, ask questions, and seek guidance so that I know my options. However, much of the time, I receive very little guidance and the doctor rushes out of the room. I know they are busy, but so am I. I take time out of my busy work schedule to go seek expert assistance from them. I don't have time to waste. I'm trying to feel better! Sometimes, they never see me again and they don't even realize they've been fired.

I had been learning about natural cancer treatments for years and had just recently learned about two nutraceuticals that were shown to detoxify the body and reduce tumors and cysts. I learned about zeolite powder and modified citrus pectin from David Wolfe. I dug in and discovered impressive research and testimonials. I also discovered the cancer-fighting properties of medicinal mushrooms from David Wolfe, as well as Paul Stamets.

I put together a program based on my research. It included modified citrus pectin, zeolite powder (clinoptilolite), medicinal mushrooms, green vegetable powder, several different berries, spinach, chard, chia, hemp, and other nutrient-dense foods. I included concentrated berry powders, including goji berry, schizandra berry, and camu camu berry from Peru, which has the highest vitamin C content of any fruit in the world.

I took a course of modified citrus pectin for two weeks. Then I switched to zeolite powder (clinoptilolite), I alternated back and forth every couple of weeks. Concurrently, I was taking reishi mushroom extract. I also drank chaga mushroom tea. All these nutritional supplements have been shown to prevent cancer cell growth and reduce the size of tumors or cysts. I also cleaned up my diet and took additional supplements. The details of my regime are described at the end of this chapter.

The day of the biopsy, I was nervous, but I knew I would receive an anesthetic. I was given an ultrasound prior to the FNA. I was so excited to find out if my nodules had shrunk. As the tech performed the ultrasound, I couldn't wait. I asked her if my nodules had shrunk, and she curtly told me, "No."

The doctor came in to perform the FNA. The needle with the anesthetic hurt, because that is a very sensitive part of the neck. Then the doctor proceeded to insert a needle about an inch deep into the front of my neck, which I felt go all the way in. I felt pressure and discomfort, not pain. He stopped, leaving the needle in, and wiggled it to get cells out. He repeated this four times. Even with topical anesthetic, it was still rough because they inserted the needle quite deeply. I was sore for about a week afterward.

Clearly, this procedure is easier for people with large or even small nodules that are readily accessible. The doctor can easily extract cells from nodules that are right there. Mine on the other hand were less than one millimeter, so he was inserting the needle deeply into my neck and moving it around. He was "digging" because as I found out later, he was unable to get ANY cells. They were THAT small!

Nodules Disappeared

I waited with bated breath for about a week and half to get the call with the results. I was so anxious to know if my program was successful. When the doctor finally called with the results, he said **they were unable to get enough cells out of the nodules**. Thus, they were unable to test for cancer.

He sounded quite grave and disappointed. He asked me if I wanted to repeat the test and he sounded unsure about why he was asking. What logical person would repeat a test where a doctor jabbed a needle into their neck four times, an inch deep, just to fail the mission? Weren't they thorough enough the first time?

Obviously, **they didn't get any cells out because the wonderful natural medicine I took was successful!** Clearly, it was not necessary to repeat the test, because the doctor probably still would not be able to get enough cells out of such a tiny nodule. Of course, they would certainly be able to bill me, wouldn't they?

Dr. CuttThroat then explained, almost as an afterthought, that the larger nodule they originally measured at 12 x 12 mm had shrunk to 0.8 x 1.0 mm! I'm not sure if the measurement is taken in two different ways (length by width or diameter perhaps), but my original ultrasound report said the larger nodule was 1.3 cm. It's only a 1 mm difference so if we go with the original report, it shrunk by 12 mm total (from 1.3 cm or 13 mm to 1.0 mm) or maybe it shrunk by 11 mm. Either way, it's significant. The smaller nodule was undetectable! My response was, "Hell yeah!" I was totally thrilled! That's what I was waiting for! That's what it was all about! For whatever reason, he didn't share in my joy.

> **Large nodule shrunk from 12 x 12 mm -> 0.8 x 1.0 mm**
>
> **Small nodule was UNDETECTABLE**

I told Dr. CuttThroat happily that my program worked and offered to send him my protocol in email. He declined. He said, "You can send it regular mail if you want." What a nerve! He did not seem to be interested in helping his patients. He sounded so disappointed! Maybe he had been planning a trip to Aruba with the profits from slicing my neck open and taking my precious thyroid gland out. For what other reason would he possibly be upset and disappointed after a patient healed herself of a potentially cancerous condition? A normal decent human being would be impressed and congratulate me, and perhaps suggest that I follow up in a year. He did no such thing. Dr. CuttThroat was SO fiiiiirrrred!!!

And no, I did **not** snail-mail him anything because I presumed he was uninterested in using it to help anyone. While I was very grateful that my nodules shrank, I was shocked and disappointed not only by the behavior of Dr. CuttThroat, but also by the lying ultrasound tech. I asked her if my nodules had shrunk, and she said that they were still there. How could she not see that they had shrunk to a twelfth of their original size? I suspect she couldn't see them at all. Perhaps the biopsy wasn't even necessary because the nodules were so small. After repeating the ultrasound, they didn't even consider canceling the FNA procedure. After all, they billed my insurance about $3000 for it. I paid $250 of that. To be fair, this is their day-to-day work. It probably doesn't even enter their consciousness that a patient could cure themselves prior to their test.

Still Gone After 10 Years

I was thrilled that my program worked, and my efforts are still working. I no longer fear cancer.

I had a recent ultrasound in November 2022. The ultrasound report states, "Stable thyroid nodules—no follow-up is recommended." The report explains at the bottom that an FNA biopsy is recommended if nodules are greater than 15 mm and that a follow-up ultrasound is recommended if nodules are greater than 10 mm. It says on the report that mine are less than 5 mm, and that no follow-up is required!

I am sharing this story to inspire hope and show how disease can be reversed, something many doctors would tell you is impossible. After all, even after I succeeded and offered the endocrinologist my protocol, he wasn't interested.

Working with your Doctors

I recommend that people use this information while working with their own health professionals. However, I suggest that people facing chronic health issues should find a doctor trained in functional medicine or complementary medicine (ACAM certified). Some things are covered by health insurance, and some aren't. You can see an Osteopathic Doctor (OD) or a Naturopathic Doctor (ND) and ask them to evaluate your lab results and diagnostic tests that your primary physician orders, which are covered by insurance. I have not experienced any of my doctors working together, but they are very open to reviewing any diagnostics from other physicians. My primary physician is a DO and practices complimentary medicine. I also see an internist that is integrative and very knowledgeable about supplements and exercise, and I have an eye doctor and an OB/GYN that are integrative. If you can't find any integrative physicians in your area, there are many functional medicine doctors that meet virtually with patients. Form your own team of health practitioners that are agreeable to complimentary medicine. You can even go a step further and find experts that are knowledgeable about the latest advances in holistic or complementary medicine.

Both allopathic (mainstream) and holistic medicine have their strengths and benefits. Many chronic conditions, including autoimmune diseases. are treated more effectively when allopathic and naturopathic or functional medicine are combined.

We need multiple approaches for optimal results. We should all have access to "integrative medicine."

My Original Thyroid Nodule Protocol

Described below is the protocol I put together in 2013 based on the information available to me at the time. I stand by this protocol and think it can help people to shrink their thyroid nodules because it worked beautifully. However, after a decade of continuous healing, growth, and education, I have enhanced this protocol and expanded on ways to heal the various root causes of Hashimoto's. This program can be customized for people based on where they are in their journey. Dosages, for example, can vary based on the brand, and the person's weight, age, and sensitivities. Still, it is important to document the original successful protocol in this body of work. You will learn much more later in this book about things you can do to elevate your healing higher and higher.

Original Thyroid Nodule Protocol from 2013
Modified citrus pectin—For the first two weeks, I took six capsules (5 g), three times a day. I alternated every two weeks with zeolite powder.
Zeolite powder (clinoptilolite)—For the second two weeks, I took two capsules of zeolite powder every six hours. Later, I changed to the powder and added 1 tbsp to my smoothie each morning. I alternated every two weeks with modified citrus pectin.
Selenium—I increased my intake by eating three or four Brazil nuts several mornings each week. I also took one 200 mcg capsule of selenium each evening with dinner.
No gluten and dairy.
Reduced sugar intake.

Original Thyroid Nodule Protocol from 2013

Daily breakfast porridge of pumpkin seeds, chia seeds, flax seeds, raw cashews, blueberries, coconut flakes, and cinnamon (recipe shared below).
Daily smoothie with coconut water, scoop of green powder (such as Tonic Alchemy by Dragon Herbs), blueberries or banana, stevia, one dropperful of goji berry, schizandra berry, and reishi mushroom extracts. Sometimes, I would change it up a bit. Sometimes, I would use different fruit or add fresh spinach leaves. Often, I would add a teaspoon of goji berry powder or camu camu berry powder.

The smoothies were delicious and energized me through the whole morning and early afternoon.

Note: The protocol described above only includes the additions and changes to my standard daily supplement routine, not my entire daily protocol. I was still taking vitamin D, magnesium, and other supplements daily.

Skeptics may say any one of these things did it alone, or that it was pure coincidence, but I believe that when you are facing a serious health condition, why take chances with only one option? And why allow a physician who has a financial interest in your treatments to interfere with your decisions in choosing alternative approaches?

Hit it with all you've got! Give yourself the best nutrition you can. Add more new superfoods into your diet, especially berries, avocados, and mushrooms. Be sure to get enough healthy fats, such as coconut oil, avocado, and quality extra virgin olive oil (but not too much). Nuts and seeds can be consumed in reasonable amounts for healthy snacks or incorporated into recipes. Chapter 11 contains more detail on diet. Invest in a high-quality water filter and an excellent blender for super smoothies. Small changes over time can add up to big benefits. Your body has an innate ability to heal itself given the proper tools and nutrition.

After my program was successful, I applied to be a citizen journalist for *Natural News* hoping that I could share my protocol. After I was accepted, I wrote an article entitled "Woman shrinks thyroid nodules with pure nutrition, not meds." It was published December 17, 2013. It provides a short overview of my condition and includes an overview of the regimen I followed.

Most of the feedback on my story was excellent and supportive. A few commenters however, thought I was complaining too much or exaggerating about the soreness I experienced after the needle biopsy procedure. One said it was very misleading because she didn't have any pain at all. Some internet commenters (trolls) are so rude. I'm not oversensitive to pain, but I think the doctors inserted the needles more deeply into my neck because they were having trouble extracting any cells. In my case, the nodules were practically nonexistent at 0.8 mm by 1.0 mm. It would be easy to extract cells from a nodule that is easily found. Just imagine a nodule that is one or more centimeters. It would be easy to insert a needle into it and extract cells, probably in one try. I spoke the truth and simply shared my story. It is not in my nature to exaggerate or mislead anyone. On the contrary, all I want to do is help people.

Porridge Recipe
This is a tasty creamy and nutritious breakfast porridge. **Ingredients:** • 1 tbsp each of pumpkin seeds, chia seeds, and flax seeds • 2 tbsp coconut flakes • ½ cup raw cashews • 1 tsp cinnamon • Pinch of salt • Stevia or monk fruit to taste • ½ cup blueberries
Directions: • Blend the pumpkin seeds, chia seeds, and flax seeds, coconut flakes, cashews, salt, and cinnamon. • Add boiling water and stir. • Add sweetener of your choice to taste. Stevia or monk fruit are good choices. • Top with blueberries.

Types of Thyroid Nodules

Thyroid nodules are solid or fluid-filled lumps within a thyroid gland. Most thyroid nodules aren't serious and don't cause symptoms. Most nodules are noncancerous, or benign. Around 50 percent of people have a thyroid nodule by the age of 60.[16]

The vast majority of thyroid nodules are benign but should be checked to make sure they are not growing. Occasionally, some nodules become very large and can be felt and seen on the neck. In these cases, if you press on the windpipe or esophagus, it can cause shortness of breath or difficulty swallowing. According to the radiology center that ran my recent ultrasound, any nodule over 1.5 cm (15 mm) should be biopsied.

Thyroid nodules are categorized into the following types:

Thyroid Adenoma

Thyroid adenomas are benign growths of normal thyroid tissue. No treatment is necessary if they are not causing discomfort and compressing your neck. Follow-up ultrasounds are performed to monitor them periodically.

Toxic Adenoma

Toxic adenomas are thyroid adenomas that secrete excessive amounts of thyroid hormone. This causes hyperthyroidism (an overactive thyroid). Symptoms can include unexplained weight loss, nervousness, tremors, sweating, or rapid or irregular heartbeat. Malignant cancer from a toxic adenoma is very rare (between 1 and 8 percent).

Thyroid Cysts

Thyroid cysts are fluid-filled nodules in the thyroid. Pure thyroid cysts are usually benign (non-cancerous).

Goiter

Any enlargement of the thyroid gland is referred to as a "goiter." Goiter can be caused by iodine deficiency or by Hashimoto's. A goiter can occur in a thyroid that is producing too little hormone (hypothyroidism), too much hormone (hyperthyroidism), or the right amount of hormone (euthyroidism). A goiter indicates there is a condition causing the thyroid to grow abnormally.[17]

Iodine deficiency is one cause of goiter. The body needs iodine to produce thyroid hormone. If you do not have enough iodine in your diet or live in a region where the soil is low in iodine, the thyroid may grow larger to try to capture all the iodine it can. Treatment is unnecessary for goiters unless the goiter is causing compressive or hyperthyroid symptoms.

Multinodular Goiter

A multinodular goiter is an enlarged thyroid that contains multiple nodules. These nodules are almost always benign. They only require treatment if you are experiencing compressive or hyperthyroid symptoms, or if one or more of the nodules is suspicious for thyroid cancer.

Thyroid Cancer

According to the Johns Hopkins Department of Otolaryngology and Head and Neck Surgery, more than 95 percent of thyroid nodules are benign (non-cancerous).[18] However, it is wise to be aware of the risks of developing thyroid cancer and ensure you are getting the proper tests so that if it does develop, you can catch it early. You should also be aware of the over-diagnosis problem which is described below.

Thyroid cancer forms when normal thyroid cells have genetic changes that make them grow abnormally. The two most common types of thyroid cancer are papillary and follicular. They are less aggressive than the three other types of thyroid cancers (hurthle, medullary, and poorly differentiated/anaplastic thyroid cancer).

Some studies have shown that patients with Hashimoto's disease are three times more likely to develop thyroid cancer. Most thyroid cancers can be treated successfully if diagnosed early. Sadly, thyroid cancer takes the lives of approximately 2,000 people annually. However, the death rate has remained at a low level over the past few decades, while the number of cases diagnosed has gone up (due to increased testing).

In comparison, the following are the estimated deaths annually per cancer type according to the American Cancer Society:[19]

- Breast cancer: 43,700
- Digestive system: 172,010

- Respiratory system: 132,330
- Brain and nervous system: 18,990
- Genital system: 69,660
- Lymphoma: 21,080
- Leukemia: 23,710

Overdiagnosis of Thyroid Cancer

Benjamin Franklin said, "If everyone is thinking alike, then no one is thinking."

Did you know that there is scientific evidence of overdiagnosis of thyroid nodules and thyroid cancer, leading to unnecessary surgeries?

Overdiagnosis is defined as finding cancer that will never cause any symptoms and will not affect the quality of life and the overall survival of a person. It has been reported that **overdiagnosis accounts for up to 60–90 percent of all cases of thyroid cancer** in various countries.

After removing the thyroid gland, it is tested for cancer. It is estimated that about 10,000 Americans needlessly have their thyroid glands surgically removed every year because of thyroid nodules or growths that were **wrongly classified** as cancer.[20] Just imagine if patients with thyroid nodules received health coaching and started dietary changes and supplementation with selenium, zinc, vitamin D, modified citrus pectin, etc. Thousands of people could be spared unnecessary surgery, harmful side effects, and a lifetime of thyroid-replacement medication.

The American Cancer Society clearly states that the increasing rate of thyroid cancer is due to detection during imaging tests (such as CT or MRI scans) that were ordered for other medical problems. The testing technology today is *so* precise that it detects small thyroid nodules that might not have ever been found. Many of these tiny nodules would never have caused any problems.[21] Due to overdiagnosis, **healthy people have unnecessary diagnostic tests and treatments, including surgery,** which puts people at risk of complications and causes the unnecessary anxiety of facing a cancer diagnosis.

According to a study in Finland, occult papillary carcinoma (OPC) can be considered a normal finding which should not be treated when found incidentally (such as during other scans). This study indicates that unnecessary thyroid removal operations can be avoided by identifying small OPCs (less than 5 mm in diameter) as an occult papillary tumor rather than carcinoma.[22]

Cancerous Nodules?

Were my thyroid nodules cancerous? They may have been, but there is no way of knowing because the attempt to extract cells during my biopsy failed completely. Why? Because I shrunk them down to almost nothing. So, do I want to know if it was cancer? No. Not really. I was curious but I was concerned that I would experience a strong fear reaction. They were virtually gone in any case. As long as they didn't come back, I was not going to live in fear. Everything turned out fine. However, even if it was cancer, I have confidence that I have the ability to prevent and heal that as well.

Remembering Jill

I have had family members and friends with cancer, and most of them were too afraid to do anything other than what the doctor said. One of my dear friends, who I met in 2021 at a crystal and gem show, suffered with cancer five times. I called her my Jilly Jill and we met while reaching for the same crystal. She was 75 and she told me some of her story the first day we met. We hit it off immediately and it was no coincidence that we met. I gave her a big hug, along with some pain cream and sacred skin oil. We kept in touch and spoke often. We were on the same spiritual wavelength and we laughed together so much. I wish I had more time with her, but I'm grateful I was able to spend time with her before she moved to Florida to be cared for by her daughter. I coached her and helped her lessen her pain and symptoms. I made her homemade Essiac tea and delivered it. I also ran my Rife machine on her remotely and she said she experienced immediate pain relief. Her pain was severe, and I was extremely happy and grateful that the remote Rife therapy worked so well for her. After moving to Florida, her new oncologist gave her chemotherapy one more time and then stopped because it was too hard on her. She had become very thin and frail and soon after the treatment, she went into hospice. She passed on to the other side on April 10, 2023. I miss her but I'll always remember her smile, her kindness, her giggles, and our conversations full of fun, laughter, spirit, and inspiration.

There are many alternative treatments for cancer and other diseases but unfortunately, they are often suppressed and discredited. I have studied natural cures for cancer since the 1990s. There is so much hope. I practice preventative measures such as taking anticancer supplements, oxygenating my body, taking care of my mental health, using frequency healing, and eating foods rich in cancer-fighting antioxidants. There are many advanced treatments and more are being developed all the time.

It is very empowering to have the confidence to heal myself and not to be reliant on mainstream physicians. They are limited by a system controlled by large powerful companies and institutions. I have read that medical doctors face the threat of losing their medical license if they break protocol. They are "inDOCtrinated" to deny the power of holistic medicine. They must treat patients with the tools in their toolbox, which are essentially drugs and surgery. I acknowledge that, but I don't have to put myself at risk and follow their protocols. I evaluate their suggestions, and I ultimately make my own protocols. I may take medication after reviewing the side effects, but if I am aware of effective natural and safe alternatives, I prefer to choose those instead or at least try them first.

Risks of Thyroidectomy

You may be reading this book because your doctor advised you to remove all or part of your thyroid. I strongly believe that removing body parts should be avoided if at all possible. In my opinion, it is logical and sensible to try safe natural medicine to resolve problems before reaching such a dire state that surgery is necessary. Unfortunately, many people are not aware of holistic treatments and reach a point where surgery seems to be their only option.

Anytime you are considering surgery, make sure you are fully aware of the risks. Doctors often gloss over the risks of surgery. I have had doctors that didn't explain the risks of surgery to me at all. I guess it's an uncomfortable conversation for them. They usually have a staff member hand you a paper and expect you to sign it quickly. When they discuss risks, some of those risks are associated with potential mistakes that the surgeon or anesthesiologist could make during surgery. They may not want you to be aware of mistakes they could potentially make. Perhaps some of them want to instill confidence in you because people get very nervous about having surgery. In any case, you have the right to know all the risks for any procedure you have. It should be discussed. If it does not come up, ask your doctor to explain. Do your research. See if what they tell you matches with what you research.

Thyroidectomies are performed for several reasons:[23]

- **Thyroid cancer** – Cancer is the most common reason for thyroidectomy. If you have thyroid cancer, removing most or all of your thyroid is likely to be a treatment option.
- **Noncancerous enlargement of the thyroid (goiter)** – Removing all or part of your thyroid gland may be an option for a large goiter. A large goiter may be uncomfortable or

make it hard to breathe or swallow. A goiter may also be removed if it's causing your thyroid to be overactive.

- **Overactive thyroid (hyperthyroidism)** – In hyperthyroidism, your thyroid gland produces too much of the hormone thyroxine. Thyroidectomy may be an option if you have problems with anti-thyroid drugs, or if you don't want radioactive iodine therapy.
- **Suspicious thyroid nodules** – Some thyroid nodules cannot be identified as cancerous or noncancerous after performing a needle biopsy.
- **Multinodular goiter** – An enlarged thyroid with multiple nodules.
- **Restricted airway** – Airway is compressed by benign thyroid nodules.

What are the risks of thyroid removal surgery? Thyroid surgery is usually a safe operation with a low rate of complications, but all surgeries have risks.

Some of the serious risks include the following:[24]

Infection—The neck is generally a clean area and does not get infected. However, if an infection develops, drainage of the infected fluid may be needed, and antibiotics may be prescribed.

Bleeding—There is a chance of bleeding with any surgery. Average blood loss for thyroid operations is usually small and the need for a blood transfusion is very rare. However, bleeding in the neck can be potentially life-threatening because as the blood pools, it can put pressure on the windpipe or trachea which causes difficulty breathing. After overnight observation, if there are no signs of bleeding and the patient feels okay, they can go home the next morning.

Hypocalcemia—This is a common post-operative complication of total thyroidectomy. Sometimes it is difficult to correct. Hypocalcemia causes low blood calcium levels and usually results from injury to the parathyroid glands. As hypocalcemia progresses, muscle cramps are common, and people may become confused, depressed, and forgetful and have tingling in their lips, fingers, and feet as well as stiff, achy muscles. Each thyroid lobe has two parathyroid glands, which are about the size of a grain of rice. They are located near (or attached to) the thyroid gland and control the blood calcium levels. Sometimes, they are accidentally cut during surgery. After thyroid surgery, your blood calcium should be checked to ensure that the parathyroid glands are functioning normally. Calcium and vitamin D supplements are often recommended to treat hypocalcemia.

Permanent hoarse or weak voice—The symptoms of this injury vary from hoarseness to severe life-threatening respiratory distress, especially if bilateral cords are involved. Bilateral vocal cord paralysis happens when both vocal folds are unable to move. Bilateral vocal fold paralysis most commonly occurs because of a problem with the recurrent laryngeal nerve, which is the nerve which controls motion of the vocal folds. In most cases of vocal cord paralysis, only one vocal cord is paralyzed. Paralysis of both vocal cords is a rare but serious condition. This can cause difficulties with speech and significant problems with breathing and swallowing. The incidence of post-thyroidectomy vocal cord paralysis has been reported in the range of 3.5–6.6 percent of surgery patients. Fortunately, 93–100 percent of these patients made a complete recovery.

Incidence of Hypocalcemia

How common is hypocalcemia?

Total Thyroidectomy Study

From January 2015 through to April 2017, 400 patients that had a total thyroidectomy due to various thyroid diseases were studied. Hypocalcemia occurred in a whopping 257 (**64.2** percent) of patients.[25]

Note: Only total thyroidectomy patients were studied. That is at least part of the reason why the number of patients that developed hypocalcemia was significantly higher in this study compared to the California study described below.

Only 23.3 percent of the 257 patients with hypocalcemia had symptoms. However, 76.7 percent of them had *asymptomatic* hypocalcemia. That means that they did not experience symptoms, but their bodies were not making enough calcium. Is that okay because they don't have symptoms? No. Of course not! A lack of calcium increases the risk of osteoporosis, osteopenia, dental problems, depression, muscle pain, and other health problems.

This study also examined risk factors for hypocalcemia. They looked at the patient's calcium levels prior to surgery. They also looked at mistakes the surgeon might make that would increase the risk for hypocalcemia. They found a patient risk factor that can be controlled. **Patients with low blood calcium prior to surgery were at higher risk.** This is a great finding! Knowing that, patients can make sure that they have a healthy calcium level prior to thyroid surgery.

I wonder how many thyroid surgeons are warning their patients to test and/or increase their calcium levels prior to surgery? I suspect the number is low, especially since this study was conducted recently. Medicine takes a long time to catch up to the research and make changes. However, it seems obvious to me that **surgeons should ensure their patients have a normal blood calcium level before** thyroid surgery to prevent hypocalcemia.

California Study

Another study conducted over a 15-year period in California analyzed the rates of various complications and deaths in patients who had thyroid surgery in a hospital. In the California study, only 4.5 percent of patients developed hypocalcemia. All complications were examined. Why such a glaring difference?

That is because in the California study, only 40 percent of the thyroid surgeries studied were total thyroidectomies.

The researchers studied 106,773 patients who had various types of thyroid surgeries in this 15-year timeframe. Approximately 9 percent of patients experienced complications, which included both temporary and permanent types of complications.[26] The complications are summarized below:

- Hypocalcemia (low calcium levels) is a major post-operative complication of total thyroidectomy—4.5 percent of patients (4,804 people)
- Vocal cord problems include changes in voice function (dysphonia) and swallow function (dysphagia)— 1.1 percent of patients (1,174 people)
- Required a blood transfusion—0.9 percent of patients (960 people)
- Wound infection—0.4 percent of patients (427 people)
- Death—0.3 percent of patients (320 people)

The average length of hospitalization was one day. However, 41 percent of patients had to remain hospitalized for more than two days. Older patients had a higher risk of complications. Patients who had thyroid surgery done at hospitals that perform more than 100 thyroid surgeries each year were at the lowest risk. Also at lower risk were patients who had less than a full thyroid removed (partial thyroidectomy).

Takeaway

In summary, having thyroid surgery is not without risks, and the risk of hypocalcemia is significant. So if you can take steps to prevent having thyroid surgery, you can keep your precious thyroid gland and help it to function better. If you have already had it removed, there are things you can do to regenerate the thyroid. If you must have surgery, make sure you have a healthy calcium level prior to surgery.

CHAPTER 4

Of All the Doctors I've Fired Before

"You can't afford to get sick, and you can't depend on the present healthcare system to keep you well. It's up to you to protect and maintain your body's innate capacity for health and healing by making the right choices in how you live."
— Dr. Andrew Weil

Do you remember the Julio Iglesias song, "Of all the girls I've loved before"? Well, imagine that song with the words, "Of all the doctors I've fired before." I love music and I like to use my sense of humor to get me through life's ups and downs.

Doctors take a Hippocratic Oath to do no harm. I have been harmed by several doctors, and I've also been incredibly disappointed in the ineptitude of many physicians. Many of them rush through the appointment and fail to answer questions. Some doctors warn against going on the internet, but I think patients are wise to research their conditions because many doctors do not fully explain your diagnosis, risks, and long-term concerns. Some doctors I have seen have learned things from me during our visits. I am the only one paying though, and I often do not get my money's worth. I usually do my best to heal myself after taking home a copy of my lab work.

The message of this chapter is to share some entertaining stories while conveying the message that you don't have to stay committed to a doctor that is not providing you with good care. You are a paying customer, even if your health insurance pays most of it. They get paid regardless. They are not doing you a favor. They are doing their job.

They are responsible for helping you, but nothing happens to them if they don't. If they fail, you are left holding the bag. It is well worth the effort to spend some extra time and research to find the best doctors for you and your family.

Sarcasm Disclaimer

Before anyone gets triggered by my sarcasm, relax. I have respect and appreciation for many doctors, nurses, and medical establishments. While I have not had the best experiences with my chronic health conditions, I acknowledge that some people have doctors that are very effective and helpful for them. Some of those folks are happy with being prescribed the medication that doctors are supposed to prescribe as part of a standard protocol. Some of them feel better and some don't but they are not sure what else to do. Others get to a point where they feel better—not great, but better than they did before. Sadly, some of these people just don't realize how much better they can feel.

I think allopathic medicine is excellent for emergency medicine, acute care, life-saving surgeries, and many other things. However, patients with chronic conditions such as eczema, autoimmune disease, and type 2 diabetes experience better health outcomes by using functional medicine. Sometimes, our family doctors are good at diagnosis but they have completely missed it for my family on several occasions, especially when my oldest son was severely ill and hospitalized for four days. We left without a diagnosis, nor any treatment plan. In my case, I was undiagnosed for 10 years. My youngest was undiagnosed with autism for several years and he was incorrectly diagnosed as an infant with scarlatina when he actually had roseola (verified by a second pediatrician visit). He was prescribed antibiotics when he had a viral infection, and he had autism and a gut imbalance, so antibiotics could have worsened his condition instead of helping.

I personally suffer with chronic autoimmune disease and other issues, and although I have a team of doctors now that I respect and appreciate, I do most of the work myself. Often, I request the bloodwork that I think I need in order to monitor and diagnosis my conditions. My doctors regularly check my CBC, sugar, cholesterol, thyroid, liver, and other lab tests based on my history and current symptoms. However, most of them do not run labs for heavy metals, allergies, hormones, gene mutations, or Lyme tests unless I ask for them specifically.

We have a mainstream medical system that is largely focused on emergency medicine, profit-incentivized medications, and treating symptoms, but does not demonstrate strength in nutrition or preventative medicine. Most doctors are not trained in nutrition, herbology, or holistic treatments and I've found that they are not interested in discussing it unless I am speaking to an integrative physician.

Most mainstream doctors that I know of downplay any ideas that contradict their model of costly drugs and surgery. They either warn against supplements or say you can take them if you want. I was told by a gastrointestinal doctor that no one in the world has ever healed their gallstones. He wanted to remove my gallbladder. I still have it and he was wrong!

I have noticed an increase in open-mindedness in recent years with some doctors, but there are still some physicians that claim you will only make expensive urine by taking vitamins. Tell that to someone that is into urine therapy! That is a joke, but seriously, there is scientific evidence for urine therapy. I personally have not tried urine therapy and do not plan to anytime soon while I have other alternatives. Regardless, the expensive urine comment is ignorant and untrue. I've proven it wrong throughout my entire adulthood. Just as one example, the section about intravenous vitamin C in Chapter 14 references multiple studies and resources about the incredible therapeutic effects of megadoses of vitamin C. Today, IV vitamin therapy is so popular that you can schedule it online and have it administered in your home for a variety of health problems or as preventative or antiaging medicine. Many celebrities use it to recover from late nights of partying or just to stay young. But ask for it in a hospital and you get a flat "No."

Recommendations

- Always request a copy of all your lab results. They are paid for and yours to have.
- Keep a folder with your lab work for your own reference and bring it to other physician appointments as needed.
- Write down your questions before doctor visits and make sure your questions are answered before the doctor leaves the room.
- Ask your favorite doctors for recommendations to other specialists.
- Read reviews on each doctor on multiple websites.

Right to Health Freedom

Always remember that you have the right to make your own health decisions. Whether you want to take a medication, get surgery, or accept a treatment, it is YOUR decision to make. Please take some time to do your own research and educate yourself on the risks involved and search for alternatives that might be safer or more effective. It is well worth the effort. Take caution when prescribed a new medication. Don't be a guinea pig for new medications. I suggest only using pharmaceutical products that are proven to be safe with a long track record of safety. When it comes to vaccinations, I suggest that before proceeding you research the ingredients (such as heavy metals) and side effects, especially the effects on autoimmune disease. Research MRC-5 and decide if you want those cells in your body. I recommend that you research information provided by the National Vaccine Information Center, so that you can make an informed decision. You can go even further and look up the studies published in medical journals around the world.

You are Fiiiirrrred!

Okay I have not actually told any of these doctors to their face that they were fired, but they never heard from me again. And in my mind, it's just a funny way of dealing with a negative situation. I have high expectations of medical professionals. We all do. If they fail to help you, cause you pain or worsen your condition, or if they push risky treatments on you, or fail to address the root causes of your illness (especially autoimmune illness), find someone else.

Dr. Jerk

I've met some dismissive and even abrasive doctors, but Dr. Jerk wins for the most horribly behaved doctor my family has ever seen. My kids and I nicknamed him Dr. Jerk. Never in my life have I experienced such outrageous behavior from a doctor. His own staff acknowledged that he was like that. Maybe he should have undergone a detox, or some serious therapy or mood-balancing therapeutics.

Dr. Jerk was repeatedly rude to me and my children. He took my autistic son's toy out of his hand with no warning as soon as we walked in the room. He was very curt and he interrupted as I asked questions. I talk fast, but he talked so fast, it was almost impossible to take all the information in. During every visit, he walked out of the room before I finished asking the questions on my list. Yes, I made a short list (five to 10 questions) to try to keep him from leaving before I was finished. Twice he said he would be right back, and never returned.

Once, I was 12 minutes late for my appointment, and after driving 45 minutes to get there, he canceled my appointment. On one occasion, I expressed concern over my cholesterol number, and he yelled loudly in my face, "What's wrong with cholesterol?" and changed the subject before we could discuss it and then quickly exited the room. I was fully aware of the debate about the link between cholesterol and heart disease and I would have liked to discuss it. His outburst was unprofessional and irrational.

He always treated me as if I was inconveniencing him with my questions. I was facing a new diagnosis of autoimmune disease and I was concerned and had questions. He answered me sarcastically and left the room in a flash. I had such high hopes when I found him because he practiced complementary medicine, prescribed vitamins, and ran extensive tests that other doctors did not, and his services were mostly covered by my insurance.

However, through my own research I have since discovered several effective nutraceuticals that he never recommended. He also ran IGG food allergy tests which were unreliable and inaccurate. He was also unaware of how badly iodine can affect a patient with Hashimoto's disease, especially when that patient is in the process of detoxing heavy metals.

There was one occasion when Dr. Jerk was so obnoxious that I got upset and broke down in tears of frustration in the chelation room. I was fed up. After that day, I never returned. Fiiiiirrrrred!

Dr. NoHelp

This doctor was our family care doctor for a while, and he was kind. Everything was okay until I had a serious problem. I developed a horrible case of eczema on my fingers. He had no suggestions to offer. He just prescribed me the steroid cream of the day. He did not offer any warnings, but he should have. That cream was only supposed to be applied for a few weeks because if used longer, it can lead to cracking of the skin. That is precisely what happened. I continued to use it for a few months not knowing the risk and my fingers started to crack open. It was painful and irritating to perform household tasks. Putting gloves on made it worse.

The itching from my eczema was so intense. I believe it goes down into the nerve level under the skin. It is like no other itch I've ever experienced. I wanted to scratch my skin off but scratching made it worse. I tried squeezing a cold washcloth around my fingers to alleviate it, but sometimes would resort to rubbing the skin and it would break and ooze and then look even worse. I tried everything I could think of to calm the itching including:

- No jewelry
- Running cold water on it
- Icing it
- Using cortisone cream (Benadryl cream seemed better than other brands for me)
- Applying a variety of eczema creams (I made one made myself which worked the best for healing the skin but only partially calmed the itching)

- Placing my hand in cold watery oatmeal. This helped more than anything.

I had all my amalgam (mercury fillings) removed. I cut dairy out of my diet and that helped somewhat but did not cure it. I went back to Dr. NoHelp three years after originally asking for help with eczema. I mentioned to him that cutting dairy from my diet helped me. He quickly agreed, saying, "Oh yeah. Dairy avoidance can help." Oh really Dr. NoHelp? Why didn't you say that three years ago? Why would you let me suffer for years? And why didn't you warn me about the skin cracking side effect? Then you have the nerve to bill me for that visit? This was after I had visited him with a written list of all my symptoms. I spelled it out for him. I knew I had a thyroid problem way back then. I had a list of about 15 symptoms. No help at all. I sent his bill back along with my list of symptoms and a letter, explaining that I had laid out all the issues I had, and I did not receive any help. In fact, the only thing done for me was the prescription of skin-cracking cream. I kindly asked them to waive the bill and they did. Fiiiiirrrrred!

Dr. TrancePharm

As I mentioned in Chapter 3, I visited a doctor that I call Dr. TrancePharm because his eyes were closed as I was telling him about my symptoms, including how I felt depressed, fatigued, and breaking out. He leaned back with his eyes closed and chanted quietly, "Prozaaaaaac . . . birth controooool . . ." I was sitting across from him observing him in his trance-like state just saying the names of medications, knowing full well I did not plan to take any of them! I knew then that even if they helped, they were only band aids to treat the symptoms, and would not cure me because they had nothing to do with my root causes. He was too strange, slow, and sleepy for me. Fiiiiirrrrred!

Dr. Synthroid

My former primary care doctor referred me to an endocrinologist after running a standard thyroid panel on me with normal results. I had to insist on thyroid antibody tests after doing my research and being fully confident that I had a thyroid problem.

I then visited a young lady who was an endocrinologist, and she ran a full thyroid panel. She did not share my lab work with me. She simply said she was going to "put me" on levothyroxine and to come back in six months. She didn't know I had already done my research on thyroid medications, and I did not wish to take Synthroid (levothyroxine), but she left no room for discussion. I asked for a copy of my lab results on the way out. I only had one abnormal result. My TPO antibodies were elevated. They were 144. Normal would be less than 35.

During my short visit with this doctor, I attempted to engage her in a discussion about nutrition and asked her questions about iodine. She just smiled placatingly at me and didn't offer one bit of advice or information. Instead, I saw her writing on her pad and I could SEE what she was writing. I asked her point blank. "What are you writing? 'Consistent with Hashimoto's.' Is that my diagnosis?" She quietly admitted that it was. She was NOT going to tell me my diagnosis! In addition, she prescribed a drug that does not consistently work, and certainly doesn't address autoimmune disease. She also neglected to discuss any other medication options and didn't tell me anything about my diagnosis. Fiiiiirrrred!

Dr. CuttThroat

Dr. CuttThroat was the second endocrinologist I visited. I went to see him after my ultrasound results revealed that I had two thyroid nodules. He said that my nodules were suspicious because of their hypoechoic pattern and uneven edges, which increases the odds of thyroid cancer.

I asked him what would happen if it was cancer. As I described in Chapter 3, he did not respond verbally. He made a **cut your throat hand-motion** across his own neck. No words. That was highly unprofessional and insensitive. Thus, the name Dr. CuttThroat. I was kind of shocked and didn't respond to it at the time. I was worried about having cancer and I didn't want to have surgery. Use your words and be kind Dr. CuttThroat. Fiiiiirrrrred!

Dr. Rookie

I had read several books about bioidentical hormones, and I was impressed with the work of Suzanne Somers, not to mention how amazing she always looked. I wanted to get tested because I suspected I had a hormone imbalance. I found a doctor specializing in this and when I called, she answered the phone and spent a good 20 minutes talking to me. I thought that was unusual but nice. When I visited her office, it became clear. No one was there. She must have just started her practice. She tested my blood, and it turned out my progesterone was extremely low, instead of a whole number, it was a fraction and she seemed very alarmed. My T3 level was also low.

Both times I went to her office, I was the only patient there. It was empty. I noted that she had two very young girls working for her. She prescribed Armour Thyroid 60 mg and a shot of progesterone. One of the girls, whom I presumed was a nurse, administered a painful progesterone shot in my upper arm. I was in severe pain for the next three days to the point where I was unable to use my arm.

The only good thing about this experience was that I was prescribed Armour desiccated thyroid hormone. I took 60 mg of Armour Thyroid for one year. It didn't help me feel any better, but it seemed to alleviate my constipation which had been an ongoing problem. That alone made it worth it. After a year of this medication, I started having heart palpitations. That was alarming. I weaned myself off the medicine and later followed up with a different doctor.

I decided not to go back. I didn't just fire her because of the painful shot but that was the main reason. I also didn't feel comfortable being one of her first patients. I had been sick for too long. I needed an expert. Fiiiiirrrred!

Dr. PushyPillPusher

I visited a female gynecologist that did a very comprehensive exam which included an aggressive questioning session about my sexual partners. I had just recently gone through a divorce. I wasn't sleeping around. She lectured me sternly about condoms and HIV. She told me that when I want to have sex with a new partner that we must both get full testing done including HIV testing, and even after a negative result, we must use condoms for a full year and then get retested. Her attitude was not caring. It was aggressive and uncalled for. She had no right to question me that way.

I went to her for a gynecological checkup, and she had a detailed intake form. I was open about my symptoms. I already knew at this point that my thyroid was off, based on what my body was telling me. That was likely related to my symptoms. However, she pushed hard for me to take birth control pills and go on Prozac. Neither of those drugs would have helped my thyroid autoimmune condition. This was after my divorce, and naturally I was depressed but I did not want to take medications with side effects. I knew I could safely use holistic medicine instead and continue to get to the root cause of my symptoms. Fiiiirrrrred!

Dr. BoneCrusher1

I had neck and back pain in my early twenties when I started working at a desk all day. I also suffered whiplash after a car accident, so I began seeing a chiropractor regularly. He had actually visited our company to seek out patients. I bought into the spiel of getting regular adjustments when I saw my crooked spine on an X-ray. However, one day, instead of pushing down in the middle of my back, he pushed down very hard directly on my right shoulder. I felt like he crushed it and like something went wrong. It wasn't like a normal crack. For the rest of that day, I felt a deep, aching constant pain traveling down from my shoulder through my whole arm. My arm was weak, and I was very concerned. I called him and he denied any culpability. He had the audacity to suggest it was caused by using my mouse! I guess they learn in medical school never to admit to harming anyone. I was so frustrated because I know my body and I felt the injury happen right beneath his hands. Then I felt the continuing pain for the rest of that day. I used my mouse every day, so his defense was ludicrous. I told them not to send me a bill and he and his wife/assistant both yelled at me. I was shocked. I told him he would be lucky if I didn't sue him. Fiiiirrrrred! And I did not get a bill.

Dr. FeckMyShoulder

In 2019, I joined a new company, and I began to experience a great deal of mental and emotional stress. I had an extremely heavy workload, and I was being harassed by a couple of female employees including my managers which made it impossible to avoid. The emotional impact of this situation took a major toll on my health and triggered my autoimmune disease to flare up. I became so inflamed, that I developed severe shoulder pain and sciatica.

Meanwhile, my mother was chronically ill and suffered several falls. She didn't want to move in with me, so I was helping by hiring people to assist her. Several of them did not work out and one of them stole from her and manipulated her feelings, which caused a lot of stress for my mother and I. I was driving back and forth from New Jersey to Connecticut to help her every few months but less often than I would have liked because I was in a lot of pain.

When I started this job, I was in remission and feeling well physically and emotionally. The stress, physical pain, and emotional and mental anguish I experienced manifested in severe physical illness. I was also diagnosed with a stroke in my left eye, and I had to start getting injections in my eye every couple of months. The excruciating pain in my right shoulder continued to worsen. I couldn't even lift a coffee cup to my mouth without severe pain. It started with an "impingement" and led to major surgery. I tried physical therapy, but the pain continued to worsen. I finally went to a pain management center. I was not willing to take any opiates, especially after witnessing the toll opiates took on some of my loved ones. I was looking for a long-term solution.

Dr. FeckMyShoulder was a lovely young lady and I liked her very much. She was kind and knowledgeable and I put my trust in her. I brought my mom to see her and she helped her by injecting medicine into her arm, which helped unfreeze her shoulder and allowed her to eat with both hands. That alone improved her quality of life. I'll always be grateful to her for that. She also sent white roses when Mom died which was very kind.

She assured me that they would not bill me for anything over what insurance paid. That influenced me to go along with the procedures they recommended. Besides, I was desperate for relief. I could not reach up for anything with my right arm. First, she did an ablation, burning the nerve in my neck that led to my shoulder. That gave me complete pain relief! It lasted for only three months and the nerves grew right back. When my nerves grew back, I had electric shock-like pains in my neck and the pain returned.

Next, she suggested a procedure called a "tenotomy." They put me under general anesthesia and used a needle to extract what she said was "inflamed tissue" from my shoulder. I did not experience any pain relief. A few short months later, I was turning my steering wheel for a sharp curve, and I felt my rotator cuff tear. It was a pain that I had never felt before. I sat in the car holding my shoulder and praying and talking to my mother, who had recently passed.

A few days later, I was tossing a heavy pillow across my bed, and I felt another tear. A third tear happened later after Dr. Bonecrusher2 used extreme force on my shoulder (story below). I had a full rotator cuff tear and a tear in my bicep and labral as well.

After my rotator cuff, bicep, and labral tore, the pain management practice that thinned out my tendon tissue advised me to get surgery. When I asked the surgeon if the thinning of the tissue led to the tears in my tissue, guess what he said? Oh no, of course not. Again, I think they are trained not to admit culpability. Dr. FeckMyShoulder, you are a lovely lady and I forgive you because I know you were trying to help me, but you are fiiiiirrrrred!

Dr. StemCellFail

I was afraid of having the shoulder surgery because I had heard about how difficult the recovery can be. I had read about stem cell therapy, and I had some successful Protein Rich Plasma (PRP) treatments previously, so I believed in its potential. Dr. StemCellFail had given me PRP treatments, so I drove 90 minutes to his new office, gave him the MRIs, and he professed confidently that his treatment would work. The procedure cost $10,000 out-of-pocket. He started by performing liposuction on my flanks to extract stem cells from my fat for the injections. The nurse then prepared the injections while I waited. I noticed that she was *not* wearing gloves. Soon after, Dr. StemCellFail injected my shoulder, knees, and neck without any anesthesia, and it was incredibly painful.

I went home and I waited to feel better. Weeks later, I went for two expensive follow-up PRP injections which Dr. StemCellFail had neglected to mention was part of the protocol after the surgery. He did not tell me I needed additional PRP treatments until *the day of* the stem cell procedure. That was sneaky on his part and a huge shock to me. I had to put another huge chunk of money (~$4,000) on my credit card.

Nothing. It didn't work. In fact, soon afterwards, warm, inflamed red blotches appeared in the areas of the injections. I was alarmed and I went to the ER to get checked out. I wanted to make sure I didn't have blood clots. Thankfully, it was not blood clots. It was cellulitis. The ER prescribed antibiotics. I called Dr. StemCellFail and I sent him pictures. Guess what? He didn't admit any fault—of course. He blamed me and said it was probably bug bites. It looked nothing like bug bites. I took photos of the affected areas (my knees and shoulder) and it looked nothing like bug bites. They were large red raised blotchy patches of skin and they were warm to the touch. I had not left my bedroom and I didn't have any bugs visiting me there! I was bed-ridden, recovering from those painful injections and the cellulitis infection, and I never left the house. Thus, bug bites were a ridiculous suggestion. Ludicrous and lame. Complete failure and waste of money. Fiiiirrrrred!!!

Dr. BoneCrusher2

After the failed cell stem surgery, I went to a local chiropractor who I had visited from time to time when I had back pain. He thought he could help me. I was alarmed how rough he was with me. He was digging his fingers into my flesh all around my injured shoulder and it was incredibly painful. He claimed he was breaking up the inflamed tissue. On my last visit to him, he pushed down extremely hard directly on my torn rotator cuff. It killed! I couldn't believe he did that! I said, "Why would you push directly on my injury!? It is just going to inflame it more." Less than an hour later, I was home, and I dropped something on the floor. I reached down to pick it up and felt my shoulder tear for the THIRD time! I was done. At that point I gave up and resigned myself to the fact that I needed to go through the surgery. Later, I wrote Dr. BoneCrusher2 a letter and I explained to him what happened, and strongly suggested that he should be more careful with people, especially senior citizens because he could seriously injure people. I told him not to bill me and he did not. He also did not admit culpability, but he did apologize. I knew him for years so that was better than the others, but still, he is fiiiirrrrred!

Major Surgery

After the stem cell surgery being a complete failure, and after Dr. Bonecrusher2 worsened the injury, I felt like my arm was falling off. I had a constant gnawing pain and sharp stabbing pain when trying to lift anything. I had to get the surgery. I was afraid of a long recovery and my fears were well-founded. I had a long recovery ahead of me.

I had major shoulder surgery in September 2020. We shall call the surgeon Dr. Stiches. He used two anchors to repair my rotator cuff and one anchor to repair my bicep. He removed a bone spur and repaired the labral with stitches. He also removed inflamed and arthritic tissue. I am grateful to the surgeon because he repaired the damage and answered all my questions and concerns. He communicated with me through email and I appreciated that. I learned that the torn tissue could atrophy, and if you wait too long, it might not be repairable. I'm glad I went through with it. However, Dr. Stitches gave me four large stitches that look like Xs, one of which came open a few times and continued to itch. I wish he would have done a better job with finer stitching.

Although it has been over three years since the surgery, I still have continuing pain and burning periodically in the middle of my upper arm. I asked Dr. Stitches about it and he said it may be radiating down from my shoulder. I'm not sure if I believe that. I have found evidence that damage to the deltoid muscle has been reported after rotator cuff repair procedures. The area of pain is my deltoid muscle. I know he meant well, but I wonder if he was aware of this potential error and did not want to admit that he may have nicked my deltoid. In any case, it's not worth having another surgery to fix it. Why would he admit to potentially making a mistake? Especially after the tenotomy creating the need for the surgery in the first place. For these reasons, he's fiiiiirrrrred!

I did 10 months of physical therapy three times a week and exercised at home on the off days. I had a frozen shoulder the whole time. The therapists were perplexed as to why it wasn't loosening up. They were cranking my arm up and down trying to get me to have full motion. It wouldn't budge.

This is where Hashimoto's comes in. They did not seem to understand (even though I told them several times) that I experience more inflammation than the average person because I have autoimmune disease. Finally, we agreed together to take a break from physical therapy to see if it would calm down. After stopping physical therapy, my arm relaxed, and I was able to gain full motion after a couple months. It was a very long and slow healing process.

I tried several different natural anti-inflammatories during this ordeal. CBD and turmeric did not help my pain and stiffness whatsoever. The only things that truly helped were ice packs, carbon 60 (C60), and reducing sugar. What is C60? Learn more about this impressive natural medicine in Chapter 13.

Takeaway

Suffice it to say, everyone makes mistakes and no one is perfect. It is easy to be intimidated by people of authority but remember that you are a paying customer. I want your takeaway from this chapter to be this: Your time is precious and your health is paramount to your enjoyment of life. You deserve the proper diagnosis and treatment in a timely manner for your conditions. Sometimes, you may have to dig and push a little to ensure you receive the proper care, whether it be from mainstream or alternative medicine providers.

CHAPTER 5

Eight Keys to Healing Hashimoto's

"The doctor of the future will give no medication, but will interest his patients in the care of the human frame, diet, and in the cause and prevention of disease."
– Dr. Andrew Weil

Your thyroid health is critical for your metabolism and overall health. There are several key factors necessary to treat and reverse hypothyroidism. This chapter gives you an overview of the keys to healing hypothyroidism and Hashimoto's disease. The following chapters will describe in more detail how to address these keys to healing.

Key 1: Proper Diagnosis

Finding a doctor that is aware and astute enough to run lab tests that help him or her to assess your condition accurately is an essential first step.

It is critical for you and your physicians to understand approximately 90 percent of hypothyroidism is caused by Hashimoto's autoimmune disease.[27] The most common tests for diagnosing Hashimoto's disease include thyroid antibody tests and thyroid ultrasounds.

You may receive a thyroid ultrasound as part of an overall physical exam or because your doctor orders one based on your symptoms. Ultrasounds provide high-resolution images of your thyroid that can help your doctor assess the health of your thyroid gland.

The following two antibody blood tests should be run for you by your doctor to determine if you have Hashimoto's autoimmune thyroiditis. After being diagnosed with Hashimoto's these tests should be run regularly to help manage your condition.

- Thyroid Peroxidase Antibody (TPO)
- Thyroglobulin (TG)

Any doctor can order these tests. If they don't want to run it, I would go somewhere else. My antibody tests have been ordered not only by an endocrinologist, but an osteopath, internist, optometrist, and even my gynecologist! If you really don't have a choice and your doctor won't order these tests for you, you can order them yourself through various labs online for a reasonable cost. Some insurance plans reimburse patients for online lab tests. Some doctors also consider a diagnosis of thyroid nodules on an ultrasound an indication of Hashimoto's disease even if antibodies are not elevated.

In the early stages of Hashimoto's, up to 80–90 percent of people will have TPO antibodies, TG antibodies, or both. However, the TSH, Free T3, and Free T4 levels are typically normal. **That is why many people go undiagnosed for years**, and when a doctor finally does diagnose them with Hashimoto's, they are often told to wait and watch, and may be offered antidepressants for their misery, or birth control pills for their hormone-related problems.

Many patients are prescribed the most common thyroid medication, levothyroxine (Levo-T, Levothroid, Levoxyl, Synthroid, Tirosint, or Unithroid). It's a man-made (synthetic) version of what a healthy thyroid makes. There are several natural versions of thyroid hormone medication, such as WP Thyroid, Nature-Throid, or Armour Thyroid, which are brand names for a natural form of thyroid hormone made from the dried thyroid glands of pigs. These medications contain all four thyroid hormones (T1, T2, T3, and T4). Beware of thyroid medications that contain ingredients with gluten. Dr. Izabella Wentz, PHARMD, warns that many prescription medications contain gluten in some of their ingredients and can sabotage your healing.[28]

Many doctors ignore the fact that 90 percent of hypothyroidism cases are caused by Hashimoto's autoimmune disease. Hashimoto's disease leads to hypothyroidism, not the other way around. The cause is rooted in autoimmunity. Currently, there are no treatment recommendations or guidelines in the world of conventional medicine to address the immune system's attack on the thyroid gland. The predominant focus of mainstream physicians is to restore normal thyroid hormone levels. Thyroid medications help to increase your T3 and T4 thyroid hormone levels, but do not lower antibodies or correct the autoimmune condition. The thyroid will continue to be attacked and slowly destroyed.

Prescribing thyroid hormone is the well-documented, established protocol for thyroid disease across all major medical resources.

I interviewed an internist who told me that many doctors do not tell patients they have Hashimoto's disease because they do not know how to treat autoimmune disease. If they don't know how to treat it, they should at least tell the patient about their condition so that they can seek alternatives. This system is completely failing people with autoimmune diseases. Some autoimmune diseases may be better researched and treated than others, but at this point, Hashimoto's is a poorly and ineffectively treated condition. When autoimmune disease is left unbalanced, the body is at higher risk for the development of other autoimmune conditions.

I have a **suggestion for doctors**, especially endocrinologists. Consider **simply prescribing Low Dose Naltrexone (LDN)**. It would be a great start. LDN is covered in Chapter 7.

If you have elevated TPO or TG antibodies, the root causes of your autoimmunity must be determined and treated or eliminated. If you focus solely on the thyroid and not the autoimmune problem, the healing is far less likely to be successful. In the chapters that follow, you will learn how to manage autoimmunity and recover your health.

Key 2: Identify Root Causes

There are many root causes that can lead to autoimmune disease, and Hashimoto's in particular. Not everyone's root causes will be the same, as we are all individuals and have our own histories, genetics, diets, habits, lifestyles, and environmental exposures.

However, according to Dr. Alessio Fasano, director of the Center for Celiac Research and Treatment at Massachusetts General Hospital, three main factors must exist for autoimmunity to develop:

1. A genetic predisposition
2. Intestinal permeability (also known as "leaky gut")
3. Triggers (infections, food sensitivities, etc.)

The most common root causes of Hashimoto's disease include the following. Chapter 6 provides detailed information about each of them:

- Genetic weakness or mutations
- Heavy metal toxicity
- Environmental toxins
- Allergens
- Stressful events
- Neck injury
- Poor gut health
- Bacterial Infections
- Viral infections (past or present)
- Parasite infections

Medications and Illnesses that Affect your Thyroid

There are several gastrointestinal disorders that prevent your cells from absorbing thyroid hormone. These include H. pylori (Helicobacter pylori) infection, lactose intolerance, undiagnosed celiac disease, atrophic gastritis (inflammation and thinning of your stomach lining), and malabsorption in the small intestine.

There are also some medications that have negative effects on thyroid health. Some medications destroy thyroid cells, some interfere with thyroid hormone production, some affect immune function, and some can trigger Hashimoto's disease. Some medications are made with fillers that contain allergens (such as lactose or gluten), or chemicals that can negatively impact your thyroid.

Thyroid pharmacist Izabella Wentz advises thyroid patients to avoid these nine medications:[29]

- Lithium (Mood stabilizer)
- Amiodarone (A-Fib medication)
- Fluoride and medications made with fluoride
- Birth control or hormone replacement therapy using oral estrogens

- Proton pump inhibitors (PPIs) such as Prevacid and Prilosec
- Interferon (cancer treatment)
- Accutane (acne treatment)
- Iodine (see Chapter 12 for details)
- Botox (see Chapter 6 for details)

Root them Out

It is very important to take the time to examine your root causes. You probably have some root causes that you have never even thought about or heard of. This disease is complex, but some of the contributing factors for Hashimoto's are easily resolved and eliminated. Some take a little more time. As you address these issues, your energy and mood start to lift. Your pain may start to decrease, and your skin may improve. It is a wonderful thing to take your health into your own hands. We dig into the root causes of Hashimoto's in Chapter 6.

Key 3: Address Infections and Viruses

Infections are a hidden trigger for Hashimoto's. Most mainstream doctors do not test for these triggers, unless you ask for the tests specifically, or if you are having clear symptoms related to these infections. Functional medicine doctors are more likely to run these kinds of lab tests. It stands to reason that any type of infection is going to put your immune system on high alert. The problem is detection. Many infections go undetected either because you don't have any symptoms, or you experience common symptoms that can be confused with something else.

Bacterial infections: Several bacterial infections can trigger Hashimoto's. For example, you could have H. pylori, yersinia enterocolitica, or Borrelia burgdorferi (associated with Lyme disease).

Parasitic infections: Parasites are more common than people think. Many parasites go undetected for years as they grow and multiply, wreaking havoc in their host (you). There is a microscopic parasite that is correlated with Hashimoto's and should be ruled out. Parasitic infections can worsen viral infections and trigger autoimmune conditions.

Viral infections: There are several hidden viruses that have been associated with triggering Hashimoto's. These viruses lie dormant sometimes for years until they are reactivated due to a major stressful event or illness. Many of these viruses are in the herpes family, such as Epstein-Barr, Varicella zoster (chicken pox), cytomegalovirus (CMV), and herpes simplex viruses (HSV-1 and HSV-2). Other viruses that complicate Hashimoto's include Hepatitis C, mumps, parvovirus, rubella, Coxsackie B, and enterovirus.

Fungal infections: Fungal infections often stem from candida and include fungal skin issues, ringworm, fungal toenails, oral thrush, urinary tract infections, yeast infections, or vaginosis. Candida overgrowth causes digestive issues including bloating, constipation, or diarrhea. It damages the lining of your intestines and can lead to leaky gut, sugar cravings, allergies, chronic fatigue[30], and recurring sinus infections.[31] Major fungal infections have been shown to cause severe autoimmune disease.[32] The main causes of candida overgrowth are eating a lot of sugar or high-carbohydrate foods and taking certain medications such as birth control (pills, patches, and rings) and antibiotics.

Infections are covered in more detail in Chapter 6.

Key 4: Detox

Detoxification is very important. The thyroid is like a sponge for heavy metals, halogens, and industrial pollutants such as perchlorate. This toxic burden prevents your recovery and drags down your energy and mood. Sometimes, removing toxins such as heavy metals from your body can help you to reverse thyroid autoimmunity.

An important part of detoxification is making sure your detoxification pathways are clear by keeping your bowels moving and addressing gene mutations that affect the body's elimination pathways out of the body.

Thyroid Poisons

You must protect your thyroid from toxins that slowly poison your precious gland. Toxins can damage the thyroid and cause a disruption in the healthy normal functioning of this gland.

Chapter 6 provides detailed information and tips for avoiding thyroid toxins that are at the root of autoimmune disease including perchlorates, halogens, heavy metals, pesticides, herbicides, fungicides, and industrial pollutants. Chapter 8 explains how to detox and test for heavy metals.

Key 5: Restore Gut Health

According to functional medicine, poor gut health is the primary root cause of autoimmune disease. Intestinal permeability (also known as leaky gut) and other gastrointestinal issues are associated with the development of autoimmune disease. Many factors contribute to gut problems, including infections, food sensitivities, a lack of digestive enzymes, gut dysbiosis, and constipation. Dysbiosis is when there is too much harmful bacteria or too little beneficial bacteria.

Many people with thyroid conditions have low stomach acid (hydrochloric acid, or HCl), which breaks down protein. If you don't break down proteins efficiently, it can lead to a depletion of amino acids, zinc, iron, B vitamins, and other nutrients that are obtained from eating proteins.

See Chapter 6 to learn more about the causes of gut problems, and Chapter 10 for a guide to heal your gut.

Key 6: Fill Nutrient Deficiencies

Most people with Hashimoto's have micronutrient deficiencies. While it's challenging for many of us to get the nutrition necessary to prevent health problems caused by nutrient deficiencies, it is even more difficult for people with Hashimoto's or hypothyroidism. Some factors slow down or prevent the absorption of nutrients in the cells of people with hypothyroidism.

The active form of thyroid hormone (T3) reaches every cell in your body, from your muscles to your brain cells. Having the proper amount of T3 helps to increase your metabolism, your mood, and your energy. Your body needs healthy amounts of the following **minerals** to produce an adequate amount of thyroid hormone that your body can use.

- **Magnesium**: Helps to reduce Hashimoto's antibodies. Low magnesium leads to low selenium.
- **Selenium**: Helps to reduce Hashimoto's antibodies and converts thyroid hormones to their active state. Low selenium is associated with low COQ10 levels (which can affect heart health).
- **Zinc**: Helps to convert thyroid hormones to their active state and triggers your hypothalamus' thyroid hormone receptors.
- **Iron**: Converts iodide (from your diet) to iodine to form thyroid hormones and helps convert thyroid hormones to their active state.
- **Iodine**: Used by the body to produce thyroid hormones. See Chapter 12 for clarification on the iodine debate and a warning about supplementing with iodine.

Protein Intake

Protein intake and assimilation is also very important for Hashimoto's because it helps with gut health and immune function. It can also help prevent and reduce problems such as muscle weakness and blood sugar disfunction. Your body has storage facilities for fat (adipose tissue), but not for protein. Too bad we can't switch that around and just have our fat disappear every day! You must take in quality protein (and essential amino acids) every day, through your diet or with supplements.

Causes of Nutrient Deficiencies

Nutrient deficiencies can occur if you eat nutrient-poor foods, or don't eat enough food. However, even if you eat an organic, nutrient-rich diet, many factors can put you at risk for micronutrient deficiencies. These include:

- Inflammation from infections or food sensitivities
- Low amount of stomach acid
- Calorie restriction
- Fat malabsorption
- Imbalance of gut bacteria
- Deficiency in digestive enzymes causing poor breakdown of nutrients
- Some medications
- Alcohol consumption

Seven Common Nutrient Deficiencies in Hashimoto's Patients
1. Vitamin D
2. Vitamin B12
3. Selenium
4. Zinc
5. Magnesium
6. Iron/ferritin
7. Thiamine (Vitamin B1)

These nutrients are described in detail in Chapter 13.

You should consult with a well-versed health professional to customize your doses based on your lab work, preferably with an integrative physician, functional medicine doctor, or naturopathic doctor.

Key 7: Add Immune Modulators

Immune system modulators help to calm your immune system down when it's attacking, or boost your immune system when needed to fight infections. The following are immune system modulators:

- Medicinal mushrooms (see Chapter 13)
- Immune modulating herbs (see Chapter 13)
- Low dose naltrexone (see Chapter 7)
- Stem cell therapy (see Chapter 16)

Key 8: Restore Adrenal Balance

Does any of this sound familiar? If so, you may be experiencing adrenal fatigue.

- You wake up and have trouble functioning without plenty of caffeine.
- You have a boost of energy during the early part of the day.
- Your energy levels crash around 2:00 p.m., rise around 6:00 p.m. and fall again around 9:00 p.m.
- Your energy increases again around 11:00 p.m.

The adrenals are two small glands (on top of each kidney), that release hormones such as cortisol and adrenaline when you are under stress. These hormones help to balance stress, calm inflammation, regulate blood sugar and body fat, control potassium and sodium levels (impacting blood sugar), influence sex drive, and support anti-aging.

Cortisol is known as the "stress hormone." Many people with Hashimoto's have low cortisol levels. Symptoms of adrenal fatigue include the following.

Symptoms of Adrenal Fatigue		
Chronic fatigue	Autoimmune conditions	Hypothyroidism
Depression	Irritability	Anxiety
Brain fog	Hormonal imbalances	Hair loss
Weight gain	Insulin resistance	Cravings for salt and sugar
Sleep issues	Muscle loss	Low libido
Inability to cope with stress	Light-headedness	Skin issues

What Causes Adrenal Fatigue?

Stress is the most common cause of adrenal fatigue. Constant activation of the stress response puts a demand on the adrenals to produce cortisol.

The eight top causes of adrenal fatigue are:

1. Mental and emotional stress—Feelings that create stress, such as anxiety, grief, fear, guilt, overwhelm, etc., create the need for more stress hormone.
2. Inflammation—Chronic inflammation can be caused by irritable bowel, injuries, joint pain, obesity, toxin exposure, infections, or reactions to food or drink. Cortisol is released to calm the inflammation.
3. Long-term consumption of too much caffeine—Excessive caffeine from coffee, tea, or energy drinks can drain your

adrenals. It depletes your body of nutrients essential to your adrenals, such as vitamin B1, calcium, and potassium.

4. Lack of exercise—You need exercise so your body can release built-up stress.
5. Chronic lack of sleep—Sleep deprivation can be caused by insomnia, unusual schedules or work shifts, sleep apnea, and other health issues that affect sleep.
6. Nutrient deficiencies—Your adrenals need several nutrients to function effectively. These include vitamin C, vitamin B1, zinc, magnesium, potassium, and vitamin D.
7. Chronic infection—Underlying infections can drain the adrenals. You may have contracted a virus years ago and thought it was resolved, but that virus can be reactivated during a stressful time. This can happen with infections such as Epstein-Barr, cytomegalovirus, and Lyme disease.
8. Metabolism and glycemic imbalance—Up to 50 percent of people with Hashimoto's have huge blood sugar spikes when eating carbohydrates which causes lots of insulin to be released, followed by a big drop in blood sugar (hypoglycemia).

Diagnosing Adrenal Fatigue

This topic is debated among conventional and holistic experts. Conventional blood tests do not catch adrenal problems unless they are very severe. People are considered to either have normal endocrine function or total endocrine failure (that is, Cushing's syndrome or Addison's disease).

People that experience chronic stress and adrenal imbalance usually cannot get any help from mainstream doctors, because their cortisol levels are usually in the normal range on blood tests.

Adrenal fatigue, known as "hypoadrenia" is the middle ground syndrome recognized by functional medicine practitioners. They diagnose it by observing symptoms at specific times of the day when energy spikes and drops. Many natural medicine practitioners with experience in a clinical setting know that hypoadrenia is a real problem and is associated with several complications.

Fortunately, holistic treatment for adrenal fatigue is effective and beneficial to your health, despite the diagnosis or lack thereof. In Chapter 13, you will learn about ways to restore your adrenal health, including information about therapeutic herbs that nourish and restore your adrenal glands.

Next-Level Healing

After you go through the initial steps of addressing your root causes and adding missing nutrients, you can elevate your health to a whole new level.

You don't have to do all the things in this book at once, but over time, you can boost your health and your mood by trying new things. Keep an open mind and a positive outlook. Remission is definitely attainable! I have reached remission several times. I have been triggered out of remission. I have made leaps and bounds by taking courses of many different herbs and nutraceuticals, getting various alternative treatments, and addressing my inner spiritual and emotional health.

Healing happens with time. It took many years to develop autoimmune disease and it won't resolve overnight. However, you can transform your health as myself and many others have done, layer by layer, over time. When you take a big step in your journey and you feel a huge positive difference, rejoice! But don't stop there. It can get better and better. Our bodies have a tremendous capability to heal.

In the coming chapters, you will learn how to address your root causes, resolve nutrient deficiencies, heal your gut, remove toxins, shrink and prevent thyroid nodules, restore your energy, and much more. Let's go!

CHAPTER 6

Identify Root Causes of Illness

"If someone wishes for good health, one must first ask oneself if he is ready to do away with the reasons for his illness. Only then is it possible to help him."
— Hippocrates

The causes of Hashimoto's disease are very wide-ranging. There are many contributing factors, and it varies for each person. Keep in mind that finding your root causes is a journey. You may address some problems and then still experience symptoms. You might feel much better after resolving one or more of your root causes, but remember, you could potentially feel even better! The aim is to rule out ALL root causes so you can feel your best and lower your risk of other health problems. As you work through addressing your unique triggers, you will likely feel better in increments.

The following are all potential causative factors for Hashimoto's disease. The first three conditions must be present for autoimmunity to develop.

Causes of Hashimoto's Disease	
Genetics and family history *	Nutrient deficiencies
Intestinal permeability (leaky gut) *	Radiation exposure
Environmental triggers *	Excessive iodine intake
Severe stress	Excess estrogen levels
Chemical toxicity (heavy metals, pesticides, pollutants)	Medications
	Dental procedures
Viral Infections	Gut problems, including IBS and infections
Bacterial Infections	Food sensitivities
Parasite Infections	

One of my reasons for writing this book is to save you time, money, and suffering. I suffered for more than a decade unnecessarily because of doctors that were not aware of the root causes of this disease and not interested in discussing them. It's maddening to think of how many thousands of dollars I spent on doctor visits, lab tests, treatments, books, supplements, specialty foods, classes, summits, and conferences.

I have met many women who encountered similar frustrating experiences. One woman told me that her endocrinologist said, "You know, there is no cure for Hashimoto's." He prescribed her Prozac, and she suffered horrible side effects, including thoughts of suicide. Sadly, many physicians are unaware of how to help their patients and thus ignore their patients' complaints or prescribe medications to treat symptoms. Many of these medicines fail to help and often introduce more imbalance and cause harmful side effects. I say to these doctors, "Do us all a favor and step aside. Stop taking away hope. Stop doing harm. Refer your Hashimoto's patients to a functional medicine doctor or an integrative physician. Thank you."

Lab Test Guide and Recommendations

To discover your root causes, you must seek out the specific tests you need for proper diagnosis and root cause assessment. Most of these tests are covered by insurance but some are not. Parasite testing for example is typically not covered, but it's inexpensive ($60–$150) and I cannot stress how important it is to eliminate parasites, even the microscopic or intracellular parasites.

As a patient, whether you are paying out of pocket or your insurance is paying, you are a paying customer. You deserve to get a proper explanation of your diagnosis. You also deserve a copy of all your lab work, scans, and test results.

Always ask for a copy and keep a folder with your medical records. This is very helpful not only for your understanding of your health history, but also when you visit other practitioners. With Hashimoto's disease, you need a team of doctors. Our current mainstream medical system is divided by body parts or systems. You may have a primary physician, endocrinologist, internist, gynecologist, gastroenterologist, rheumatologist, neurologist, and dermatologist. You may also decide to work with a naturopath, health coach, herbalist, Reiki practitioner, or massage therapist. I personally do not see an endocrinologist because in my experience, they only focus on the thyroid and not the autoimmune disease.

Having your health records in hand is helpful not only to share with practitioners, but to dig in and do your own research after doctor visits. Doctors are often in a hurry and do not take the time to explain all your lab results. Ask questions. I recently asked my doctor to come back into the room as he was running out the door and I still didn't get a chance to voice all my concerns. I find it works better if I have the questions written down on paper and hand it to him or her. Then they go through the list. It just takes a little preparation.

If you go see a doctor that rushes you out too quickly and writes you a prescription and says, "try this," ask them to explain why they prescribed that drug. Is it because of the formulary they are supposed to follow? **A "formulary" is a list of drugs covered by a given health insurance plan.** Don't hesitate to ask questions. It may be a recommended drug on the formulary, but it might not be right for you. What are the side effects? Does the drug contain gluten? Will it interact with anything you are taking? Are there other options? Consider asking for a medication that has a long track record of success instead of being prescribed a new potentially risky drug.

In general, the following types of testing help you to find your root causes:

- Comprehensive thyroid testing
- Nutritional deficiency testing
- Adrenal (cortisol) testing
- Heavy metals testing
- Gut health testing
- Food allergy testing
- Gliadin, IgG, IgA (gluten antibodies)
- Infections (Lyme, bacterial, viral, and parasite tests)
- Genetic testing

The table that follows includes the top 10 tests used to evaluate your thyroid health. Note that reference ranges and optimal ranges differ depending on the lab.

Test Abbreviation	Test Name	Reference Range	Optimal Range
TSH (lU/mL)	Thyroid Stimulating Hormone	0.45–4.5 Best result is around 1.00	1.0–2.0
T4 (ug/dL0	Total T4	4.5–12.0	6.0–12.0
T3 (ng/dL)	Total T3	71.0–180.0	100.0–180.0
FTI	Free Thyroxine	1.2–4.9	1.2–4.9
fT4 (ng/dL)	Free T4	0.82–1.77	1.0–1.5
fT3 (pg/mL)	Free T3	2.0–4.4	3.0–4.0
rT3 (ng/dL)	Reverse T3	9.2–24.1	9.2–18.0
TPO	Thyroid peroxidase	<35 UI/mL	<2 IU/mL
TG	Thyroglobulin	<35 UI/mL	<2 IU/mL
TSI	Thyroid stimulating Immunoglobulin	0–140	<140

First Sign of Thyroid Disease on Lab Work

Elevated thyroid antibodies (TPO and TG) are usually the first indication of a thyroid problem on lab work. They are certainly not the first indication symptom-wise, however. I knew I had a thyroid problem based on my symptoms years before lab work provided hard evidence. I asked at least 10 different doctors over the span of 10 years to test me for thyroid illness. I didn't know at the time to ask specifically for antibody tests.

Keep in mind that the presence of elevated thyroid antibodies means that active destruction is happening in your thyroid gland. Imagine all the people that suffer needlessly for years because their doctors do not order the proper tests. I'll bet it is in the millions. How about some preventative measures? How about proper testing based on symptoms? We hear a lot of talk about preventative medicine and screening—here is a perfect opportunity to practice it and help countless people.

Call To Action

Improve Diagnosis and Early Detection of Hashimoto's Disease

Thyroid antibodies can be elevated for five, 10, or even 15 years before an abnormal TSH level is revealed on a lab test.

This information, combined with the high prevalence of thyroid disease, leads me to suggest that thyroid antibody lab work should be added to routine screening tests, especially for women of child-bearing years.

Early detection of Hashimoto's disease could make a colossal impact to improving women's health, especially if combined with a functional medicine approach to treatment.

Why aren't the thyroid antibody tests run earlier? Is the established protocol to wait until the problem is serious enough to prescribe medication or even to warrant surgery?

Thyroid Hormone Conversion

If you have low T4 or T3 hormone levels, you may be prescribed thyroid medication. Sometimes they result in relief and sometimes they do not. Many synthetic thyroid hormone medications have T4 only and rely on your body to convert the T4 to the usable T3 hormone. Levothyroxine (Synthroid) has been the most prescribed drug for several years. In 2021, it ranked as the fourth highest selling drug.[33]

Some people choose to take natural (desiccated) sources of thyroid hormone. I've read that the desiccated thyroid medications are a better choice than the synthetic medications because desiccated thyroid medications, such as Armour, WP Thyroid, and Nature-Throid, have the full range of thyroid hormones, including T4, T3, T2, and T1. This is helpful when people cannot convert T4 to T3 efficiently.

What interferes with your body's ability to convert T4 hormone to T3 hormone? There are several factors. Some of them include low progesterone, heavy metals or pesticide toxicity, medications, radiation, nutrient deficiencies, stress, and excess iodine.[34] It is thought that T4 can get converted to rT3 instead of T3 under these conditions. The rT3 is considered an inactive compound and is thought to bind with thyroid receptor sites, preventing the active form of T3 from being used. The rT3 test is not typically used by mainstream physicians but integrative physicians use this test to assess if a patient is properly converting T4 thyroid hormone and to monitor improvement.

Thyroid Stimulating Hormone (TSH)

As described in Chapter 1, there are five stages of Hashimoto's disease and TSH may be mildly elevated in stage three, and more elevated in stage four. Although getting diagnosed in stage four is late, it is still possible to reverse the disease process.

Within this chapter, you will learn the root causes of Hashimoto's disease which happen to also apply to many other illnesses. Resolving these problems can greatly improve your condition and significantly improve your overall health.

Epstein-Barr (EBV)

Epstein-Barr, also known as EBV, Mono, Mononucleosis, glandular fever, and human herpesvirus 4, is a member of the herpes virus family. It is one of the most common human viruses. More than 95 percent of the world's population is estimated to be positive for EBV.[35] If you have an EBV test, the results will most likely indicate that you had a previous EBV infection. EBV is found all over the world. Many people are infected with EBV during childhood. After you have contracted EBV, the virus remains latent (inactive) in your body for many years after the initial infection. It can awaken and reactivate itself at any time. When reactivated, it can spark the production of thyroid antibodies and cause multiple debilitating autoimmune symptoms.

The EBV virus has become more problematic because it has mutated over the last few decades. It causes problems with people's health that they may not be aware of, including thyroid problems. There is strong evidence suggesting a link between EBV and thyroid autoimmune disease. A 2015 Polish study found the Epstein-Barr virus in the thyroid cells of 80 percent of people with Hashimoto's and 62.5 percent of people with Graves'. The control population (people without any thyroid disease) did not have **any** EBV cells in their thyroid gland.[36] A more recent study in 2020 also found higher levels of EBV in patients with Hashimoto's.[37]

Is the Epstein-Barr (EBV) virus linked to thyroid nodules? In his book, *Medical Medium Thyroid Healing* (2017), Anthony William explains that thyroid nodules form in order to wall off and protect the thyroid tissue from the EBV virus. William states that EBV cells remain in your liver, and that your body stores a memory of all your past infections. This makes sense, as we develop immunity from infections we have had in the past. The problem with EBV however, is that these viral cells can grow in number, and can cause health problems during times when your immunity is low.

You can take steps to reduce the number of EBV cells by avoiding the foods that these living organisms consume and thrive on (such as gluten, dairy, and eggs) and by taking antiviral supplements and eating antiviral foods. See Chapter 7 to learn about antiviral protocols. You might think it's strange when William says viral cells survive by eating certain foods but consider this: Chicken eggs are used in scientific experiments to grow bacteria and viruses in petri dishes. In fact, **flu vaccines have been grown in chicken eggs for over 70 years**. So yes, viruses eat to live!

After having read almost all of his books, I can confidently tell you that Anthony William has a lot to offer. He has immense knowledge of health conditions and his gifts as a medium have been shown to be real many times. His book *Liver Rescue* is especially fascinating. Our livers are incredible organs. They perform thousands of functions. It is in our livers where some level of pathogens such as Epstein-Barr, Lyme, strep, herpes, and other viral cells remain.

Having his books is a treat. They are so well-crafted and beautifully enhanced with vibrant illustrations of foods and recipes. He also includes supplement protocols for many conditions at the end of his books.

Gut Problems

Gut problems are caused by many different factors. Many people have imbalances in their biome such as small intestinal bacteria overgrowth (SIBO), dysbiosis, enzyme deficiencies, low stomach acid, leaky gut (intestinal permeability), and lack of beneficial bacteria. Other problems include infections like H. pylori, parasites like Blastocystis Hominis, or food sensitivities (especially to gluten, dairy, and soy).

Beware: Some popular weight loss medications (semaglutides) that help with weight loss cause some serious gut problems, including gastroparesis. This is a condition that causes delayed emptying of the stomach, which leads to constipation, nausea, vomiting, distended stomach, heartburn, impaired absorption of nutrients, and poor glycemic control.[38] You may be desperate to lose weight, but the long-term effects of these new medications are unknown and the risks are serious. I would advise listening to many doctors that are sounding the alarm.

Chapter 10 includes a six-step guide to healing your gut.

Infections

Patients with Hashimoto's can experience many gut-related infections, which can negatively affect their immune system. The following infections should be ruled out.

Yersinia entercolitica

The most well-researched gut infection is Yersinia entercolitica. This is a bacterium you can get from eating raw or undercooked pork. Yersinia antibodies have been found in Hashimoto's and Graves' patients. Treating this infection has helped some people reach remission of Hashimoto's and Graves' disease. On the other hand, a person that just takes thyroid medication and doesn't treat this infection may experience a worsening of their condition that could lead to the development of more autoimmune conditions. You can be tested for Yersinia antibodies through a blood test. The antibiotic medication doxycycline, and herbal protocols including berberine, oregano oil, and wormwood, can eliminate Yersinia effectively in many cases.

Enterococcus gallinarum

The NIH published a study in 2018 where scientists found that a gut microbe, enterococcus gallinarum, triggered an autoimmune disease in mice that are prone to such autoimmune diseases. The mice were treated with a microbe-specific treatment, and it stopped the autoimmune issue. The researchers also found the same microbe in the livers of people with autoimmune diseases, but not in those without autoimmune disease.[39] This is more evidence that addressing gut infections can help treat those with autoimmune disease.

Helicobacter pylori (H. pylori)

Several autoimmune diseases have been linked to H. pylori infection. Some studies did not show any correlation between H. pylori infection and Hashimoto's while others showed a clear association where anti-H. pylori IgG levels were higher in patients with Graves' disease and Hashimoto's than in the control groups.[40] Most people don't realize they have an H. pylori infection because they never feel sick from it, but it's worth ruling out whether you have symptoms or not. It's a simple breath test.

Leaky Gut

Thanks to the pioneering research of Dr. Alessio Fasano, leaky gut is established as one of the primary triggers for **all** autoimmune disorders, including autoimmune thyroid disease. Normally, your intestinal lining acts as a barrier between your intestines and your bloodstream. Leaky gut occurs when your intestinal lining becomes permeable, thus allowing potentially harmful substances such as bacteria, toxins, and undigested food particles to travel freely through your bloodstream.

Gluten is one of the main causes of leaky gut. When you eat foods or drink beverages with gluten, your body may produce zonulin, a chemical that causes the tight junctions of the intestinal walls to break open and stay open.

Leaky gut can also be caused (and worsened) by:

- Gut infections such as candida, parasites, or SIBO
- Medications such as antibiotics, steroids, or birth control pills
- High-stress levels

As long as your gut remains leaky, the threats just keep on coming and your immune system stays on high alert to neutralize the threats. Your immune system may start attacking your own tissue by mistake. Leaky gut triggers widespread inflammation and leads to various conditions, including autoimmune diseases, brain fog, migraines, food sensitivities, autism, skin conditions, and chronic fatigue.

Even if you do not have a gluten intolerance, when you eat gluten and you have leaky gut, your immune system begins to attack your thyroid because your thyroid cells have a similar molecular structure to gluten. This is called molecular mimicry. One molecule "mimics" another. If left untreated, you risk developing other autoimmune diseases and potentially developing more serious gut issues. Read about how to heal leaky gut in Chapter 10.

Parasites

Parasites are a scary topic for some, but it is an absolute must for you to eliminate any parasites in your body. Parasites are a root cause for many health problems including the development of autoimmune disease and cancer. Some parasitic infections can reach the brain and cause seizures, epilepsy, and even blindness if left untreated.[41]

Contrary to popular belief, parasites do not only exist in tropical or developing countries. They are found worldwide and affect all kinds of people. According to many experts, we ALL have parasites. We are human hosts for many organisms. We may not have any symptoms because parasites can live in your body for years without causing symptoms. Common symptoms of parasite infections include fever, fatigue, anal itching, skin rashes, teeth grinding, weight loss, stomach pain, bloating, cramping, and neurological symptoms such as anxiety and brain fog. You can get parasites from contaminated food, water or surfaces, insect bites, and undercooked fish or meat (especially pork).

Parasites have also been shown to worsen viral infections by inhibiting the cellular process that slows down the replication of viral cells, increasing the virus's ability to take hold in the body.[42] If you unknowingly have a parasite infection, it might make it much harder for you to recover from viruses.

Parasite testing is typically not covered by insurance but it's inexpensive. You could opt to forgo the test and just do a parasite cleanse. I personally wanted to get tested to know what I was dealing with and later confirm that I had cleared the infection.

The Importance of the Stool Test

I was given a stool test kit a few years back from a chiropractor. I know. Yuck. I think a lot of us are a little put off by sending a poo sample in the mail, but it's a normal bodily function and it's something that you must do so you can figure out if you have parasites, candida, or certain infections in your stool. Like a Cologuard test, you place a sample in the container provided, label it, and drop it in the mail. My first kit was $60. I had a follow-up test done later that was close to $100. It's not terribly expensive and yes, your normal doctor should run the stool test and it should be covered by insurance, but it's not. It is rarely suggested. That chiropractor was the only one that ever recommended it to me. I once visited a gastroenterologist, and she didn't run a stool test. She wanted to do something far more invasive and do a colonoscopy on me without checking anything else. I was not even 40 yet. I asked her about leaky gut syndrome and she knew nothing. She was firrrrred!!!

The good news was that I didn't have any big scary worms. However, I DID have a microscopic parasite that has been correlated with Hashimoto's disease, Blastocystis Hominis. This parasite is known to be a causative factor for Hashimoto's. You can learn how I eliminated it and how you can heal parasite infections in Chapter 10.

Parasite tests only look for the most common parasites, not all of them. You *could* opt to forgo the test and do a parasite cleanse. There is no harm in an herbal parasite cleanse. Herbal treatment is effective and safe. However, it is good to know what you are dealing with, and then to retest afterwards to ensure you have successfully eliminated it.

Mainstream drugs for killing parasites have risks to the host—which is you. You might want to consider Ivermectin as a safe choice for *some* parasite infections. If you choose to take a prescription medicine, find out if kills both the adult worms and the eggs because some treatments only kill the adult worms and not the eggs. They may recommend repeating it periodically for newly developed worms. I prefer an herbal cleanse. Certain antiparasitic herbs have been shown to **kill the eggs and larva as well.**

Lyme Disease

According to the Lyme Disease Association, Lyme disease is found in 80 countries in the world. There are currently 195 countries in the world.

In the United States, Lyme disease is common in three major regions:

- Northeastern states from Virginia to Maine
- Upper Midwest, especially Wisconsin and Minnesota
- Northern California

An Epidemic that Worsens Autoimmune Disease

You might not think this information applies to you, but please rule out whether you have been infected with Lyme disease especially if you live any of the affected regions. Doctors do not routinely test for it in these regions unless you ask or if you present them with a bulls-eye rash.

According to the Autoimmune Association, some patients treated for Lyme disease later develop autoimmune joint diseases, such as rheumatoid arthritis, psoriatic arthritis, and spondylarthritis, and other autoimmune diseases, including **thyroid** disease, lupus, polymyalgia rheumatica, and autoimmune neuropathy. It is unknown if Lyme disease triggers these autoimmune conditions, or if Lyme disease mimics the autoimmune condition.[43] A lot of research is being conducted in this area.

According to the EPA, ticks are responsible for more than 75 percent of vector-borne illnesses reported to the U.S. Centers for Disease Control and Prevention (CDC) every year. Vector-borne diseases are transmitted to humans and animals when they are bitten by blood-feeding arthropods, such as mosquitoes, ticks, and fleas. Ticks are now an issue in 41 states (35 eastern and six western). According to the CDC, 30,000–40,000 confirmed cases of Lyme disease are reported to them annually, but they estimate the actual number of cases is probably over 400,000 because most infections are not reported.[44] If you live in any of the states affected, I suggest you take preventative measures and get tested to be sure.

Lyme Testing

The diagnosis and testing of Lyme disease is not known to be very accurate, especially in the earlier stages of the disease. I suggest you ask for a comprehensive test that includes coinfections. When you ask your primary doctor for the test, they usually run the Elisa and/or Western Blot tests. These tests detect antibodies in your blood that your immune system makes in response to the disease. Thyroid pharmacist, Dr. Wentz recommends IGeneX or Ulta Lab Tests.

Important: In the first few weeks after infection, the Western Blot test only detects Lyme about 29–40 percent of the time. The test is 87 percent accurate once Lyme spreads to the neurological system, and 97 percent accurate for patients who develop Lyme arthritis. As many as **40 percent of Lyme disease infections are not diagnosed until later stages of the disease.** If you are not diagnosed soon after being infected, this disease can progress and cause serious damage to your joints and your nervous system. Not everyone gets a bulls-eye rash—30 percent of people who get Lyme disease never get a rash. My son and I did not have a rash, but we both tested positive.

Experts acknowledge that we need better diagnostics that can detect infection at all stages of Lyme disease.

Lyme Coinfections

There are several coinfections transmitted by insects, such as bartonella, Lyme borreliosis, anaplasmosis, and babesiosis. The organisms that Lyme infection and its coinfections introduce to the human body are complex. Some are bacteria. Some are parasites. Some are viral. Just imagine what happens when these organisms intermingle in your bloodstream. They can wreak havoc with your immune system. Some of the Lyme culprits can hide out in what are called biofilms in the body. When the pathogens are hidden in biofilms, it's harder to eliminate them. There are holistic methods that can break these biofilms down.

Some symptoms of illness overlap and make diagnosis tricky, but some symptoms are more unique. For example, with a Bartonella infection, some people develop a sore behind their ear. It is persistent and takes a long time to go away. Another symptom of Bartonella is shin pain. Many illnesses cause body aches and pains, but shin pain is unique.

My elder son had these symptoms and that is why I insisted on a more comprehensive test. Initially, he did not test positive for Bartonella on the basic Lyme panel at the hospital, but Bartonella is a group of bacteria that consists of at least **37** different species or strains. In fact, Bartonella is one of the most common types of bacteria in the world. Most people know Bartonella infection as cat scratch fever, spread from a cat scratch, but it can also be spread by ticks. It can cause terrible fevers, which is what my son experienced. I diagnosed him. The doctor's failed. The ER doctors and a team of four infectious disease doctors at the hospital were unable to diagnose the problem after four days and dozens of tests. They are so fiiiirrrred! I had to pay $450 out of pocket to a Lyme disease specialist to confirm that he did indeed have a Bartonella infection, which showed up as a previous infection. He also tested positive for a previous EBV infection. Previous infections are ignored by physicians, even though some of these only show as active for a few weeks and even though many of them are latent potentially reoccurring infections that can wreak havoc down the road.

Note: Once you have suffered one of these infections, you are not immune. You can get infected repeatedly. If you are like me, and bugs find you ultra-attractive, this poses a risk. I never used to let the fear of infections from insect bites stop me from enjoying the outdoors, but I do not go hiking as much as I used to and the thought of sitting or lying down on a bed of grass is not appealing anymore!

Essential Oils Repel Insects

Essential oils serve as excellent protection. Insects are repelled by many essential oils, including peppermint, lavender, geranium, citronella, and lemongrass. In fact, many insects will NOT bite through peppermint essential oil. I make an insect repellent spray using essential oils and witch hazel. It contains distilled water, witch hazel, glycerin, and citronella, peppermint, lemongrass, geranium, lavender, and grapefruit essential oils.

My Personal Lyme Experience

I asked to be tested for Lyme disease in 2008, a few years after finding some insect bites on my ankle. It was not a bulls-eye rash, but I did have several oblong itchy blotches. Since those bites occurred, looking back, I had felt fatigued, depressed, and forgetful. It's hard to decipher if those symptoms were due to developing Hashimoto's, or if the autoimmune process started because of the Lyme disease. Perhaps it was a combination of everything.

The doctor found that I was positive for Lyme, and she said that the bands in the test results indicated that I was recently infected. I thought I had been exposed years ago. It's possible that I had been exposed repeatedly. It's also possible that this infection contributed to the development of my autoimmune condition. I used to travel to Connecticut to my father's home which was surrounded by trees and plenty of deer. I didn't feel any different after taking the doxycycline antibiotic for three weeks and she didn't retest me to ensure it was gone.

In January of 2022, I decided to get retested again for Lyme disease while seeing a Lyme expert with my son. My son had been suffering high fevers every day for over five weeks, as well as shin pain, and traveling pain. He was very ill, and we went to three different doctors and went to the ER twice. Our dog had recently had a flea infection and I wanted to be sure to rule out the possibility of flea-borne infections. The first time in the ER, they sent him home and didn't help at all. The second time, a young resident who seemed inexperienced glossed over his condition and was going to send him home again. I asked to speak to a doctor and her voice went up a few octaves and she asked me if I wanted to speak to her "attending." She might have phrased that thinking that I didn't know what an attending physician was. She was trying to get out of helping us and repeated her question a few times. I didn't want to upset her or Adam, but I did want to speak to an experienced doctor, not a resident fresh out of college.

When the attending physician came in and looked at his lab work, he was visibly concerned and immediately ordered several tests including an abdominal ultrasound. Adam had an enlarged liver and spleen. He had very low blood platelets (thrombocytopenia). He was hospitalized for four days. In the hospital, when I asked about the possibility of an infection from flea bites, the team of infectious disease doctors at the hospital looked down their noses with a placating smile and assured me that was impossible, and that fleas do not pass infections. Well, I confirmed very easily on *PubMed* that fleas *do* indeed cause infection. They didn't know what they were talking about!

The next day, we left the hospital without a diagnosis or treatment plan. We had an appointment scheduled with a Lyme disease expert. I wanted him to be tested for additional strains of Bartonella as the infectious disease team at the hospital said they could only run the basic Lyme panel which only tested for one strain of Bartonella. I was very curious about the lab test form that the Lyme specialist used. Not only did it have a section for tick-borne diseases, but it also had sections for nine mosquito-borne viruses, and a section for eight flea, fly, louse, mite, and tick-borne diseases. You see? There *are* diseases spread by fleas. The hospital doctors did not know this. Doctors do not know everything. No one does.

Dr. Lyme ran the "Genesis" test for both of us at the Medical Diagnostic Laboratories (MDL) lab in New Jersey. She also did a thorough physical examination. My son's results showed an IGG result for Bartonella infection and EBV. She said they were prior infections and did not require treatment. So, although there could be other unknown factors, my hypothesis of him having Bartonella and/or EBV was correct. I had pushed for answers because I watched my son suffer and none of the four doctors we visited or the whole staff at the hospital were able to help him. In the meantime, I was giving him an herbal protocol at home that included coated silver, vitamin C, sarsaparilla, cat's claw, and more. He also had an AO Scan remote frequency healing done for him by a kind friend. He finally started feeling better the day after the scan, about six weeks after falling ill. It's impossible to know for sure if the scan was effective in eliminating or reducing the infectious cells, but it is certainly possible.

The AO Scan technology is based on the works of Nikola Tesla, Dr. Royal Rife, Albert Einstein, and others that postulated that everything physical at its most fundamental level has an energy frequency. Pathogens, such as bacteria or parasites are destroyed when energy frequencies are directed at them.[45] Adam's fevers finally went away and over the next few months, he slowly regained his strength and healed by taking herbs and supplements and resting. He lost a great deal of weight when he was ill, but he has steadfastly worked out and followed a specific diet, and he is now 240 pounds of solid muscle and plans to compete in a bodybuilding competition in Summer 2024. I later purchased a Rife machine and I use it for many purposes, which I describe in Chapter 16.

When my Lyme test results came in, Dr. Lyme sounded alarmed when she told me my results included nine positive bands, but she didn't discuss the various "bands," that is, coinfections, that came up positive. She told me this over voicemail and never responded when I called back to speak to her. If you have five or more positive bands, it is considered a positive result. Clearly, this was a serious infection and certainly a challenge for my immune system.

She prescribed the doxycycline antibiotic. Despite numerous well-known and effective herbal and nutraceutical protocols for Lyme infections, the only tool the Lyme doctor had in her arsenal was the doxycycline antibiotic. During our visit, I asked her about some well-known herbal protocols, and she quickly dismissed the subject. As an herbalist, I was disappointed that we could not discuss herbs that have been shown to help rid people of Lyme and its coinfections.

I took the doxycycline as prescribed for 30 days. I also took antiviral herbs including Japanese knotweed, cat's claw, and sarsaparilla. After finishing the antibiotic, I did a 5-day course of Ivermectin, and for a few more weeks, I took Japanese knotweed, cat's claw, black walnut, sweet wormwood, and sarsaparilla. After 30 days, the doctor retested me to confirm the results of the treatment and she said the treatment was a success. However, she ran a different test. The first test, the "Genesis" test, was very comprehensive and tested for many coinfections. The follow-up test was the Western Blot test, which is known to be inaccurate especially in the early stages of infection. I didn't feel any different. So, I was not sure that I was cured.

I asked for a copy of the report after my visit hoping to get more detail, and they mailed me the first two pages out of six. It was a basic test that did not include the nine bands. I would have liked to view my entire report. After all, I paid out of pocket for it!

It was like comparing apples and oranges in my opinion. I thought she would have run the same test for the follow up to be sure all nine bands were clear.

In August of 2023, I requested my primary physician to run the Genesis test. This was the test that showed nine positive bands, and I wanted to be assured that all nine infections were clear. He had no problem running the test for me and I didn't receive a bill! A few weeks later, I was very relieved to learn that all nine bands were clear!

In retrospect, both times I experienced a hunch to get tested for Lyme disease, I tested positive. How do I know for sure that the doxycycline worked the first time I took it? I could have had Lyme disease affecting me for years. What impact did it have on my developing autoimmune disease?

Vector-borne diseases have more than tripled in the US in recent years according to the MDL lab that does the testing. The risk of these infections progressing is serious. Many people suffer with chronic issues due to vector-borne infections, especially those of us with autoimmune disease. I wish we could rely on doctors to do a better job diagnosing and resolving these infections.

Dangers of Heavy Metals

We are exposed to heavy metals every day in our food, water, air, and products that we buy. These heavy metals can get trapped in cells, tissues, and organs (including the brain) and over time they damage our cellular health. Acute metal poisoning is rare, but ongoing chronic exposure to metals can accumulate over time.

The heavy metals that have been shown to have the largest impact on the thyroid are cadmium, lead, mercury, arsenic, and aluminum. **Sometimes, thyroid function is restored in patients simply by detoxing their bodies of heavy metals and other toxins**. The thyroid is very sensitive to toxins so it's important to avoid any toxins that cause thyroid damage. The slow accumulation of heavy metals has been found to contribute to many diseases, including several neurological diseases, such as Alzheimer's disease, Parkinson's disease, autism, and attention-deficit hyperactivity disorder (ADHD). It also contributes to some cancers, cardiovascular diseases, kidney diseases, and reproductive problems including infertility.[46]

Although our bodies have detoxification systems that are designed to protect us, in today's world, we are being exposed to more toxins and pollutants than our bodies can handle. Some individuals can detoxify and eliminate toxins better than others. If a person has good liver, kidney, and gut health, their body may be able to eliminate many of the toxins.

However, several health conditions can interfere with the body's ability to detoxify efficiently. For example, if the person has leaky gut issues, fatty liver, blood sugar imbalance, or nutrient deficiencies, they may need extra support to eliminate toxins. Other factors that can present a challenge are mental and emotional stress, trauma or injury, a poor diet, or chronic dehydration. These issues not only prevent the elimination of heavy metals but can factor into *causing* the damaging effects of the heavy metals.

Chapter 8 describes heavy metals testing methods and how to detoxify heavy metals as well as other toxins. First, it's important to understand how heavy metals affect your health.

Mercury

One of the world's most widespread and dangerous environmental toxins is mercury. Mercury is a neurotoxin that can cause serious damage to the neurological and immune systems. There are three types of mercury that are harmful to human health:

- Elemental mercury (liquid mercury, quicksilver): Found in dental fillings, glass thermometers, electrical switches, and fluorescent lightbulbs
- Inorganic mercury: Found in batteries, certain types of disinfectants, and in chemistry labs
- Organic mercury: Found in coal fumes, some fish, and older antiseptics (germ killers like red mercurochrome)

Mercury toxicity can cause people to have depression, anxiety, panic attacks, excessive shyness, and anger issues. It can eventually lead to memory loss and dementia. Having high levels of mercury can cause damage to the brain, heart, kidneys, lungs, and immune system of people of all ages. In fact, young children and babies that are exposed to high levels of methylmercury can suffer damage to their developing nervous systems, which can lead to learning disabilities such as ADHD and autism. Mercury toxicity symptoms include:

- Memory loss, brain fog, or lack of concentration
- Anger, depression, and anxiety
- Learning disabilities

- Hair loss
- Headaches
- Insomnia
- Tingling in extremities
- Tremors or other movement disorders
- Problems with speech, hearing, vision, and balance

One of the most alarming aspects of mercury is that it quickly leaves the blood and lodges into different tissues in your body, especially the brain. Therefore, a blood test is not likely to reveal the true amount of mercury toxicity in your body. Scientists believe that shortly after mercury enters the body, it becomes tightly bound in the brain, spinal cord, ganglia, autonomic ganglia, and peripheral motor neurons. Although the nervous system seems to be the primary target for the damaging effects of mercury, it also has the potential to cause issues in other organ systems including the heart. It affects people differently depending on their genetics. Mercury toxicity is associated with many serious immune and autoimmune problems including allergies, asthma, autism, attention deficit hyperactivity disorder, eczema, Hashimoto's thyroiditis, lupus, multiple sclerosis, psoriasis, and rheumatoid arthritis.[47]

Thyroid Hormone and Autoimmunity

Mercury accumulates in the thyroid and can result in **slowed thyroid hormone production**. Recent studies showed that mercury toxicity in humans is linked to inflammation and autoimmunity, specifically to those with genetic susceptibility.[48]

Anger and Mood Disorders

Mercury toxicity is linked to anger and mood disorders. A study compared the health and moods of women with amalgam (mercury) fillings to women without any amalgams. They did very detailed evaluations and measured scores related to anger and anxiety.

Women with amalgams:

- Had higher levels of mercury in their mouths before and after chewing gum
- Reported more depression, anxiety, irritability, fatigue, and insomnia
- Scored higher on expressing anger without being provoked and experiencing more intense angry feelings

Women without amalgams:

- Scored higher on being able to control their anger and calm down
- Had higher scores on feeling pleasant, satisfied, happy, secure, and steady

This study concluded that amalgam fillings may be a causative factor in depression, excessive anger, and anxiety due to mercury affecting the neurotransmitters in the brain.[49]

Smoking Cigarettes and Neurotransmitters

Mercury is also linked to smoking cigarettes. A study found that women with amalgams smoke cigarettes significantly more than those without. There is a logical reason for this. Mercury inhibits the feel-good neurotransmitters, dopamine, serotonin, acetylcholine, and norepinephrine. Nicotine has the opposite effect on neurotransmitters. It increases levels of dopamine, serotonin, acetylcholine, epinephrine, and norepinephrine. This is one reason why some people smoke, to raise levels of those feel-good neurotransmitters. Researchers suggested that if mercury negatively affects the neurotransmitter levels, resulting in anxiety, people with amalgams might smoke more to relieve their anxious feelings.

How to Reduce Exposure of Mercury

The following describes the main sources of mercury to avoid.

Seafood: One of the biggest sources of mercury exposure is from eating large fish. There is more mercury in large fish or fish that eat other smaller fish, such as tuna, king mackerel, tilefish, and swordfish. For healthy adults, eating large fish once or twice a week is considered safe, but if you are fighting an illness or existing toxicity, you should eat it less frequently, or choose smaller fish species. One species, "big-eye tuna" known as "ahi" or "yellowfin" should be avoided entirely.

Dental amalgams: Silver (amalgam) fillings contain 50 percent mercury, and that mercury continues to off-gas and leech into the body when people eat or drink. Residues from mercury amalgam fillings are released into wastewater from clinical and home use, inevitably entering the environment. These residues transform into the most toxic form of mercury, methylmercury, which accumulates in the fish people eat. It is estimated that two-thirds of dental mercury is eventually released into the environment.[50]

Mercury crosses the blood-brain barrier in humans and destroys neurons. If you have amalgam fillings, having them removed is advised but can be hazardous unless it's done safely. If you have any amalgams, seek out a holistic dentist or one that is experienced with mercury-safe protocols. During and after having them removed, complete a mercury detox to be safe.

Vaccines: Some vaccinations contain thimerosal, which is an ethyl mercury-based preservative used in multi-dose vials.[51]

In 1999, the FDA was required by law to determine the amount of mercury in all products they oversee, not just vaccines. The FDA found that by six months of age, infants could receive as much as 75 µg of mercury from three doses of the diphtheria–tetanus–pertussis vaccine, 75 µg from three doses of the Haemophilus influenzae type B vaccine, and 37.5 µg from three doses of the hepatitis B vaccine, which totals 187.5 µg of mercury.[52] In 2001, thimerosal was removed from childhood vaccines in the U.S. However, in some developing countries, thimerosal is still in vaccines given to pregnant women, infants, and children.[53]

Flu vaccines are currently available in the U.S. in both thimerosal-free and thimerosal-containing (for multi-dose vaccine vials) versions.[54]

High-fructose corn syrup (HFCS): HFCS, used to sweeten many candies, sodas, and processed foods, can contain mercury. It is often made with "mercury-grade" caustic soda. When caustic soda is created by a mercury cell process, it's contaminated with up to 1 PPM of mercury.

Two common preservatives: Citric acid and sodium benzoate contain mercury.

Household items: Some thermometers, thermostats, button cell batteries, and energy saver lightbulbs contain mercury.

Mercury emissions: When industrial plants burn coal, oil, or wood, or when mercury-containing products and waste are incinerated, mercury is released into the air.

Aluminum

Studies show that aluminum damages the thyroid, negatively affecting iodide uptake and thyroid hormone production.[55] Aluminum has also been shown to trigger an immune response that can lead to an increase in antibodies that may attack the thyroid and potentially other tissues.[56]

We live in a time where humans are heavily exposed to aluminum. The scientific literature clearly demonstrates the negative effects of aluminum on the nervous systems of both children and adults. Aluminum exposure can lead to Alzheimer's, ALS, neurodegeneration, autism, and autoimmune disease. Aluminum is used in aluminum foil, cans, aluminum-based cookware, medications, housing materials, electrical device components, airplanes, boats, cars, and many other items.

In a study of daily and weekly intake of aluminum, the **highest amount of aluminum intake in humans was from medications, vaccines, and cosmetics (including antiperspirants).** The items that resulted in the lowest amount of aluminum exposure were water, food, cooking utensils, and food packaging.[57] Aluminum exposure from antiperspirants is through both the skin and by inhalation of aerosol sprays. Inhaled aluminum is absorbed from the nasal epithelia into the olfactory nerves and distributed directly into the brain.

Aluminum is a neurotoxin. Although it is an element found naturally in our soil, food, and water, it has no known use within the body. In fact, it can accumulate in the kidneys, lungs, liver, and brain, and can cause serious damage to the body. Aluminum has been shown to cause brain inflammation and contribute to the risk of dementia, autism, Alzheimer's, and Parkinson's disease, neurodegenerative changes, and cognitive impairment.[58] The incidence of Alzheimer's, Parkinson's disease, and dementia have increased dramatically over the last few decades.

It is very sad to see people I know suffer with dementia, Parkinson's disease, and other neurodegenerative diseases. It is something that could potentially be improved, prevented, or avoided by heavy metal detox or chelation therapy, but most people I talk to have never heard of these helpful therapies and most doctors do not recommend them.

Though there may still be debate in the scientific community, the hypothesis that aluminum strongly contributes to Alzheimer's disease is based on solid evidence. According to a review on aluminum and Alzheimer's disease on *PubMed*, immediate steps should be taken by everyone to reduce human exposure to aluminum, which may be the single most aggravating and avoidable factor related to Alzheimer's disease.[59]

Another concern with aluminum is that it builds up in your bones taking the place of calcium, which can damage the quality of your bones. People that have excess aluminum in their bones show high levels of calcium in their blood because that calcium does not get deposited in their bones. This interferes with bone mineralization, leading to osteoporosis.

How to Reduce Exposure to Aluminum

Most of us grew up using aluminum foil for cooking and food storage. We also used deodorant with antiperspirant that contained aluminum. Manufacturers make flour, baking powder, and food coloring agents with aluminum. Regular table salt almost always contains aluminum as an anti-caking agent. Other sources include cans, food containers, and cooking utensils made with aluminum. Aluminum leaches into your food especially when exposed to heat. The higher the temperature you cook with, the more aluminum leaches into your food.

- Avoid medications with aluminum. Some antacids and buffered aspirin contain up to 600 mg of aluminum per dose. If you use antacids or medications with aluminum, try to find a natural alternative, such as digestive enzymes and fresh juices with enzymes.
- Stop using deodorant containing aluminum. I tried many natural deodorants that either did not work at all or only worked for a few hours. I came up with a recipe for my own lavender cream deodorant and I'm pleasantly surprised at how well it works. There are only five ingredients and it's very simple. Simply melt coconut oil, and mix in zinc oxide, a little baking soda, plenty of arrowroot powder, and lavender essential oil. It is NOT necessary to apply chemicals and aluminum to your armpits to reduce odor.
- Avoid ingesting aluminum as much as possible. Stop using aluminum foil and any products with aluminum that touch

your food. Some people think that it's okay to store cold food in aluminum foil, but if the food is acidic or stays in the foil long enough, some aluminum may be absorbed into the food. It's best to just store in glass containers or wrap with parchment paper and then cover with aluminum or plastic wrap over the top. I personally err on the side of caution and never let aluminum touch my food.

- Use glass storage containers for storing food.
- For cooking and baking use glass, ceramic, or stainless steel pans, and use parchment paper when possible.
- For grilling use the grill as is (no foil) but when grilling smaller pieces of vegetables, use a stainless-steel grill basket.

Lead

Lead exposure has been linked to an increase in autoimmune disease, allergies, infectious disease, and cancer.[60] In fact, the immune system was shown to be especially sensitive to lead in comparison to other toxins.[61]

Lead exposure is not only from paint. It is found in many environmental and manufacturing industries such as in the production of motor and electric vehicles, ceramics, lead-glazed pottery or porcelain, and batteries. It is present in many products, including some lipsticks and dishes. Lead also exists in gasoline, drinking water, and cigarette smoke.

The main ways of lead entering the body are through inhalation and ingestion (drinking or eating). Higher exposures occur in occupationally exposed people. Lead gets distributed after exposure and accumulates in blood, bones, and soft tissues, especially the liver and kidneys. These organs are especially sensitive to lead toxicity which makes sense as they are the filters of our body.

Lead toxicity can cause various health problems depending upon the amount and duration of exposure. It can cause damage to the hematological, cardiovascular, nervous, and reproductive systems. Lead is classified as a possible human carcinogen by the International Agency for Research on Cancer (IARC). Lead exposure has been linked to increased risk of lung, stomach, and bladder cancer.

How to Reduce Exposure to Lead

- Identify risks in your home with the paint and water pipes. If you are a renter, you can request a lead inspection.
- Drink purified or spring water and always use cold water any time you use the faucet to get water for food preparation.
- Clean dusty areas with a wet cloth and mop floors regularly.
- Purchase lead-free products. Check labels on cookware, dishes, and food storage items.
- Dispose of old toys known to have been painted with lead paint.

Cadmium

Cadmium is a heavy metal that is released into the environment through mining and smelting. It is also found in cigarettes, phosphate fertilizers, sewage, batteries, pigments (coloring agents), and plastics. Chronic cadmium exposure can lead to multinodular goiter, reduce the secretion of thyroglobulin, and initiate thyroid cell hyperplasia, which may lead to thyroid cancer.

How to Reduce Exposure to Cadmium

People who work in cadmium-related industries (such as incineration of municipal waste of plastics or batteries), may inhale cadmium due to dust or fumes in the work environment.

The average person is more likely to be poisoned with cadmium from smoking cigarettes or by consuming contaminated food or water. Spinach, lettuce, sunflower seeds, potatoes, potato chips, and wheat cereal are among the top ten foods with the highest cadmium levels.

Arsenic

Arsenic is a well-known carcinogen and hepatotoxin (liver toxic). You may be unknowingly exposed to arsenic in your food, water, and even by air inhalation. People (and animals) are often exposed to inorganic arsenic through drinking water, especially in areas where water sources have higher levels of inorganic arsenic. *Organic* arsenic is found in seafood and is considered to have very low toxicity.

However, *inorganic* arsenic is present in foods because it is in the environment, especially in regions where there are substantial industrial, agricultural, or mining operations. About 90 percent of industrial arsenic in the U.S. is used as a wood preservative, but it is also used in drugs, metals, paints, dyes, soaps, and semi-conductors. High arsenic levels also come from fertilizers, animal feeding operations, copper smelting, mining, and coal burning.[62]

Inorganic arsenic is present in flour, rice, and some fruit juices. There are many products made with rice that are affected, including rice cereal made for infants.[63] Many people think that brown rice is a healthier choice, but brown rice contains more arsenic than white rice. The milling process removes the outer bran layer where much of the arsenic exists.

The Food & Drug Administration (FDA) reported in 2012 that there was too much arsenic in two foods: rice and chicken. Arsenic was introduced to chicken feed in the 1940s to improve muscle growth, fight disease, and make the meat pinker. Some of the arsenic ends up in the chicken meat, and some is excreted in the waste of the chickens, which is later used to fertilize other crops, especially rice. However, in 2014, the FDA called for the removal of three out of four arsenic-containing animal drugs from chicken feed because it transforms into inorganic arsenic.

As of 2016, arsenic is no longer to be fed to chickens.[64] I hope farms adhere to this rule. The EPA limits arsenic levels in public drinking water to 10 ppb. However, they do not have a specific limit for arsenic in foods or supplements.

Unfortunately, it's not possible to remove arsenic entirely from foods, but levels in food can be reduced. Food manufacturers are legally responsible to enforce controls to significantly minimize or prevent exposure to hazardous chemicals, including arsenic. Chronic arsenic exposure puts people at increased risk for cancer, diabetes, skin diseases, chronic cough, and toxic effects on the liver, kidney, cardiovascular system, and the peripheral and central nervous systems.[65] In fact a recent study showed that arsenic exposure is closely linked to the development of cancer especially in the lungs, liver, bladder, and skin.[66]

How to Reduce Exposure to Arsenic

Eat a varied and nutritious diet and drink clean filtered water and beverages. Choose rice from regions that have rice lower in arsenic. White basmati rice from California, India, and Pakistan, and sushi rice from the U.S. may have less arsenic than other types of rice. Choose organic products for wine, fruit juice, and rice products such as rice cereal.

You will learn how to detoxify arsenic and other toxins in Chapter 8.

Pollutants

The thyroid gland is very susceptible to damage from environmental toxins. Factors that cause a higher risk of Hashimoto's disease include **radiation exposure** (from both nuclear fallout and medical radiation), **increased iodine intake, and environmental contaminants** that affect the thyroid. Three of the most common industrial pollutants are perchlorate, polychlorinated biphenyls (PCBs), and dioxin. All three of these have been found to significantly disrupt thyroid function.

Perchlorates

The damaging effects of perchlorates on human health has been extensively researched. It is clearly established that perchlorates are toxic to the thyroid gland.[67] They inhibit the uptake of iodine and contribute to hypothyroidism.[68]

A 2010 study conducted by the David Geffen School of Medicine at the University of California, concluded that exposure to perchlorates is associated with the following:

- Reduced thyroid hormone levels
- Impaired thyroid hormone action
- Increased risk of Hashimoto's disease

The most common use of perchlorates is in propellants for rockets, fireworks, and highway flares. Perchlorates are used in the production of fireworks, explosives, munitions, matches, and some food packaging (to reduce static). It has been found in drinking water and ground water in **26 US states**. Make sure that you are drinking clean, filtered water. Also, **never use hot water when cooking**. Always use cold water.

Halogens

The thyroid gland has a natural affinity for halogens. Fluoride, chloride, and bromide are halogens, and all displace iodine and therefore can affect thyroid function. That means that if you are drinking water or showering in water that is chlorinated and fluoridated, your thyroid is absorbing those substances. This can reduce your thyroid hormone production.

Dioxin and PCBs

Dioxin and PCB exposure has been associated with reduced thyroid function and a lower level of T4 hormone. Females and older adults are more affected.[69]

Many countries monitor their food supply for dioxins. The highest levels of dioxins are found in soil and food, especially dairy products, meat, fish, and shellfish. Like perchlorate and PCBs, dioxin is a byproduct of manufacturing processes, including plastic and pesticide production. PVC in particular releases dioxins when burned. If a house burns down, and it has PVC pipes, dioxin is released.

Radiation

Radiation from environmental incidents as well as medical radiation are both linked with thyroid autoimmunity. People that receive medical radiation should monitor their thyroid autoantibodies to watch for the onset of autoimmune thyroid disease. People living in the vicinity of a nuclear power plant should keep potassium iodide on hand in case of a radiation leak.[70]

Botox

Botox, or botulinum toxin type A, is used for cosmetic purposes and some medical procedures. This toxin is from the bacterium Clostridium botulinum, which can cause life-threatening food poisoning called botulism. Botox is used in very small doses for cosmetic and medical issues.

Recently, Botox has been shown to lead to the activation of Hashimoto's. I strongly recommend that people do not get Botox injections for cosmetic reasons. If there is a medical reason, I suggest looking at all alternatives, so you do not end up worsening or adding a new autoimmune condition to your list of problems.

There was a case study about a woman with Hashimoto's thyroiditis that repeatedly experienced TSH elevations after having eyelid injections of Clostridium botulinum neurotoxin A (Botox) over a 10-year period.[71] After this, a study was conducted and published in 2010 to examine the hypothesis that a link exists between Botox injections and elevated TSH. Researchers concluded that there is a possible link between Botox and autoimmune thyroid diseases. Due to the widespread medical and cosmetic use of Botox, thyroid complications may go undetected after Botox treatment because many people receiving the injections may only have subclinical (or early) Hashimoto's disease. They may be completely unaware that they have an autoimmune condition which puts them at risk of complications and more autoimmune conditions the longer they go on without diagnosis and treatment. Remember, one of the more important parts of healing Hashimoto's is detoxing out harmful chemicals, metals, and toxins from your body. Adding more toxins in is not a good idea. I had to learn the hard way.

I personally had Botox treatments for a few years. I don't think the injections were the cause of my autoimmune disease because my thyroid problems started in my early thirties after experiencing severe stress at work, caring for my parents, and going through a divorce. I did not recognize any correlation to how I was feeling for several years. It's hard to notice connections when you are busy raising kids, working, helping family, and just getting through life. I didn't get that lightbulb moment until after I had gotten myself into remission. I was feeling great, and I got Botox not thinking anything bad was going to happen. A couple months later, I looked back in retrospect and noticed that I was feeling great until that Botox treatment.

It's embarrassing to admit that I allowed myself to be injected with Botox because for the most part, I try to live clean and avoid toxins. However, I was insecure about myself at the time. I had deep uneven brow lines, and one of my eyelids appeared droopier than the other. I also had an injury as a teenager that scarred my forehead which makes it wrinkle up in a weird way. My dermatologist was able to lift the droopy brow with the Botox treatment and completely erase the brow and forehead lines. He assured me it was safe and after giving it a try, I looked much younger, and I felt much prettier. I was in a relationship at the time where I did not trust my partner completely. He was very attractive and had perfect skin with no signs of aging. He used to tell me that he had "chances." He also told me during my pregnancy that he had cheated on every woman he was with until me. To be fair, I think the point he was trying to make was that I was so special to him, that he was faithful to me after not being faithful to anyone else. As a woman who had been betrayed before, I was instantly filled with fear and worry, thinking he wouldn't change. After that, it was hard to trust him and I lived with insecurity. The treatments helped to increase my self-confidence at the time. I continued the injections for a few years.

It was actually very fortunate that I noticed a decline after my last Botox treatment because that helped me realize that there was a correlation between the Botox and my illness. Before the last Botox injections, I had achieved remission from Hashimoto's disease with my natural treatment program. I felt energetic and happy prior to that last injection. I was raising two kids on my own and working full-time in a challenging IT career. After that treatment, I started experiencing fatigue, mood decline, inflammation, and general malaise. I never got another Botox treatment again. Sometimes you have to learn the hard way.

Neck Injury

Many people with hypothyroidism have a history of whiplash or other neck injuries. Whiplash injuries cause inflammation to the thyroid and harmful effects to the HPA (hypothalamic – pituitary – adrenal) axis. The HPA axis is a complex system that regulates our energy, hormone balance, immune function, mood, digestion, and stress response. Women are at a higher risk for neck injury because they typically have smaller muscles, tendons, and ligaments in their necks. Their cervical spine gets overextended causing stretching and tearing in the ligaments, cartilage, and other soft tissues of the neck.[72] I personally had whiplash twice and sought help from multiple chiropractors over the years which didn't seem to help. Now I stretch my neck, use a red LED light device, and get massage therapy.

In the coming chapters, you will learn how to address inflammation and support your thyroid and adrenal glands which will help to reduce the effects of whiplash injury. You will also learn how to address all the root causes covered in this chapter.

CHAPTER 7

Thyroid Healing Three-Phase Protocol

"No matter how many mistakes you make or how slow you progress, you are still way ahead of everyone who isn't trying."
— Tony Robbins

This chapter provides a high-level overview of three phases for healing and possibly achieving remission from Hashimoto's disease.

Disclaimer: This information is for educational purposes only. You must work with a qualified health professional or team of medical professionals to ensure your safety and best outcome. Always seek the advice of your medical team before undertaking a new healthcare regime.

Phase 1 – Testing and Diagnosis

Determine if you are unknowingly dealing with infections, viruses, or parasites. Once infections are resolved, thyroid antibodies should decrease because the immune system recognizes that the infection is gone. Treating infections is an important step in healing Hashimoto's. Some infections are obvious, such as a dental infection, urinary tract infection, or sinus infection. Other infections are not as apparent and should be ruled out.

Ask your medical team to test you for the following:

- Lyme disease, Borrelia burgdorferi, and related tick-borne infections (blood test)
- Latent viruses—Epstein-Barr, herpes, Cytomegalovirus, etc. (blood test)
- Helicobacter pylori (blood tests, stool antigen or breath tests)
- Enterococcus gallinarum (blood tests and other diagnostics based on patient condition)
- Yersinia enterocolitica (stool test)
- Parasites (stool test)

You must also assess any toxicity problems, allergies, and nutrient deficiencies. These all affect your immune system. Ask your medical team to test you for:

- Heavy metals
- Food allergies
- Environmental allergies
- Nutrient deficiencies

Reduce Thyroid Inflammation

Start working on lowering inflammation.

Improve diet: Avoid gluten, grains, dairy, alcohol, fried foods, processed meats, sugar (especially high-fructose corn syrup).

Reduce stress: Incorporate habits and behaviors that reduce your stress response, such as yoga, meditation, music, dancing, nature walks, whatever works for you!

Infections: Identify chronic latent infections (e.g., Epstein-Barr, herpes, parasites, tick-borne infections, mold, etc.).

Immunotoxins: Take steps to avoid exposure to heavy metals, pesticides, and chemicals.

Exercise: Exercise is a powerful anti-inflammatory and helps balance your blood sugar and hormone levels (including thyroid hormones).

Balance microbiome: Inflammation in the gut is one of the biggest sources of inflammation. It can be caused by poor diet, processed foods, lack of fiber, and toxins in food.

Nourish the Thyroid Gland

Nourish your thyroid and immune health by taking the following supplements.

Thyroid and Immune Nourishing Supplements	
Selenium Methionine	200 mcg daily
Magnesium Complex	500 mg daily
N-Acetyl Cysteine (NAC)	600–1,800 mg daily to increase glutathione
Zinc Picolinate	25–50 mg daily
Omega 3 essential fatty acids	You can take flax, wild-caught fish, or a vegan omega 3 supplement – 2,000 mg daily with food
Methylated B-complex high potency	Minimum 1 mg of methyl folate daily

Thyroid and Immune Nourishing Supplements	
Vitamin D3	Suggested dose – 5,000–10,000 UI daily with food. Your dose can vary depending on your blood test value for vitamin D. Optimal level is from **50–80 ng/mL**). Higher doses can be taken if you are severely deficient).

Note: Avoid iodine and iodide in supplements. Learn about iodine in Chapter 12.

Phase 2 – Detox, Heal Gut, and Resolve Infections and Viruses

Once you learn what current or past infections you have been exposed to, you can take action to help your body address those issues.

Viruses

Epstein-Barr (EBV) is a widespread human herpes virus, which (as discussed in Chapter 6) is a known trigger for many autoimmune conditions. More than 95 percent of adults worldwide have evidence of EBV infection.[73] EBV has been proven to be able to infect thyrocytes (thyroid follicular cells) and cause structural and molecular changes in thyroid cells. EBV is considered a human carcinogen by the International Agency for Research on Cancer and has been associated with several different cancers, including thyroid cancer, nasopharyngeal carcinoma, gastric carcinoma, and several lymphomas.[74]

Even though EBV may not be active presently, viral cells remain dormant in the body. The infection can become active again when immunity is low due to stress, exhaustion, and other reasons. The reactivated EBV virus can potentially cause an increase in thyroid antibodies and cause debilitating autoimmune symptoms. The good news is that there are many ways to reduce and eliminate EBV viral cells.

The only doctor on my team that has acknowledged this risk factor, and not brushed it off as a previous infection, is Dr. Cesar Holgado. He is a now retired OB/GYN, and he is well-versed in gut healing, autoimmune disease, and nutritional healing. In fact, he recommends the protocols from Anthony William, known as the "Medical Medium" who has published a series of books, including *Thyroid Healing* mentioned in Chapter 6. There are many foods and natural forms of medicine that can effectively reduce viral cells in the body. Chapter 9 describes safe and effective antiviral treatments.

Infections

Work with your medical team to treat any infections that your testing uncovered. If you have a parasitic infection, refer to Chapter 10 for details on parasite cleanses. If you have a bacterial infection, carefully consider if antibiotics are a good option. If you decide to take antibiotics, make sure you replenish your gut with good bacteria in between doses of the medication.

If you have a candida infection, your doctor may prescribe an antifungal medication such as Fluconazole along with a low sugar diet. My doctor warned me against antifungal medication because of the side effects. Doing too much at once can cause a "die-off" reaction and result in headaches, fatigue, nausea, brain fog, and skin rashes. That's why I prefer a more gentle, gradual, holistic approach. You can clear up candida with dietary changes and holistic treatments (including supplements, essential oils, and colonics). A low-sugar, yeast-free diet is recommended. It takes some time to work. There are also many good candida supplements available, including ingredients such as caprilyc acid, pau d'arco, oregano, triphala, anise, probiotics, digestive enzymes, and beta-glucans (from medicinal mushrooms).

Natural Antibiotics

Did you know there are natural antibiotics that do not harm the gut biome? It's helpful to use natural antibiotics as appropriate to avoid the overuse of antibiotics which can lead to candida, overgrowth of gut bacteria, and the possibility of antibiotic resistance. One of my favorite natural antibiotics is oregano oil. I buy the Telia brand from Greece. It is strong and effective. I put the drops into a capsule to avoid the strong taste. Other natural antibiotics include mega-doses of vitamin C, clove oil, colloidal silver, garlic, olive leaf extract, cordyceps, goldenseal, ginger, and echinacea. Additionally, if you have H. Pylori, Chaga mushroom can prevent stomach ulcers caused by Helicobacter pylori infection.[76] Remember that natural antibiotics kill both good and bad bacteria and thus you should replenish your biome with beneficial bacteria between doses.

Detoxing

Detoxifying your body is essential to removing what is sabotaging your health, your mood, and your energy. Chapter 8 provides guidelines for detoxing, including testing methods, what to eat and avoid, and how to manage detox reactions.

Root Cause Summary
To review, the following are all contributing factors to autoimmunity. Use the information in the upcoming chapters to help you resolve any issues in this list that apply to you. • Improve your gut health • Resolve bacterial infections • Treat past and present viral infections • Resolve parasite infections • Improve your diet • Avoid allergens and toxins • Detox heavy metals and other toxins • Treat any neck injuries

Phase 3 - Maintenance

At this point, you may have reached remission.

- Continue the thyroid nourishing supplements from Phase 1
- Maintain a healthy whole food, gluten-free diet
- Avoid foods that make you feel inflamed, puffy, or sore
- Avoid toxins as much as possible and take detoxifying binders periodically
- Pay attention to your body
- Keep your blood sugar in balance
- Nourish your mind, body, and spirit
- Make time for sleep, fun, and relaxation

Thyroid Nodule Protocol

The following is a **sample** protocol you can follow if you have been diagnosed with thyroid nodules. This protocol helped me to shrink two thyroid nodules within two months.

Nutraceutical or Food	Amount	Directions
Pectasol-C Modified Citrus Pectin	Nine capsules or 1.5 scoops of the powder form three times per day	Take 30 minutes before eating, or two hours after eating. It's best on an empty stomach. Continue for three to four weeks. Alternate with zeolite powder every couple of weeks.
Zeolite Powder Clinoptilolite	One tablespoon once or twice daily. Add to a smoothie or water	Take 30 minutes before eating, or two hours after eating. It's best on an empty stomach. The recommended dose is one-two tablespoons all at once. Drinking it mixed with water tastes chalky so I suggest adding it to a smoothie. Hydrate well throughout the day to prevent constipation.
Selenium	Eat three-five Brazil nuts daily or take one 200 mcg capsule of selenium with vitamin E on an empty stomach	Vitamin E helps with the absorption of selenium. Brazil nuts contain both vitamin E and selenium.

Magnesium	Magnesium complex 500 mg twice daily	Dosages vary depending on the formula. Taking before bedtime can help with sleep.
Vitamin D3	10,000 IU daily	Take with food.
Vitamin C	4,000–10,000 mg daily	Take with or without food.
NAC	600–1200 mg daily	Take without food.
ALA	1200 mg daily	Take without food.
Dietary Recommendations		
Stop eating gluten. Stay 100 percent gluten-free.		
Stop or reduce dairy, sugar, eggs, soy, and any foods that cause you inflammation.		
Breakfast porridge of pumpkin seeds, chia seeds, flax seeds, cashews, blueberries, coconut, and cinnamon. Recipe is included in Chapter 3.		
You can substitute with a different gluten-free, dairy-free breakfast that is rich in protein, fat, and fiber or alternate with smoothies or juices.		

Smoothie with:

- Water, herbal tea, or coconut water
- Scoop of green powder (such as Tonic Alchemy by Dragon Herbs or Bloom Greens & Superfoods). Choose a formula that includes gut-healing ingredients (such as probiotics and enzymes)
- Fresh or frozen fruit: 1 cup of strawberries, mango, dragon fruit, blueberries, or half a banana. Vary your fruit
- Herbal tinctures: 1 dropperful of goji berry, schizandra berry, and reishi mushroom or mixed medicinal mushroom extracts
- Optional: Add a teaspoon of wild blueberry, goji berry, dragon fruit, or camu camu berry powder
- Optional: Add half a cup of coconut or chick pea yogurt (non-dairy)
- Optional: Add stevia or monk fruit sweetener to taste

LDN – Medication for Autoimmune Disease

Low-Dose Naltrexone (LDN) is a low-risk, low-cost medication that is used to treat cancers, autoimmune diseases, chronic pain, and mental health issues.[77] It's the only medication I took for many years, and I still take it every night. I personally felt better on day ONE after taking it and I do not experience any negative side effects. In general terms, it works by blocking your opiate receptors while you sleep at night, which causes a rebound effect when you wake up in the morning, resulting in an increased production of anti-inflammatory endorphins. These endorphins not only help to modulate your immune system, but also help to elevate your mood and energy level. LDN can potentially double or triple endorphin activity, and that increased endorphin activity leads to better modulation of the immune system. LDN essentially tricks the immune system into healing itself.

Naltrexone, taken at a full dose of 200 mg, has been used for the treatment of addictions since 1984. LDN is a very low dose of Naltrexone. People usually start at a low dose of 1.5 mg, and then titrate up to 3 mg, and 4.5 mg. LDN has been proven to modulate the immune system and improve the conditions of people with autoimmune disease. That includes Hashimoto's disease, multiple sclerosis (MS), Crohn's, Graves', Raynaud's, Sjögren's, Lupus, and stiff-person syndrome. It also helps those with other immune system-related conditions such as HIV/AIDS and cancer. For a comprehensive list of conditions that this medication helps with, see the LDN Research Trust website.[78]

Unfortunately, LDN has been overlooked for many years despite its wide-ranging benefits. I've never met anyone that knew about this medication and that is a shame. I learned about it from Dr. Joseph Mercola. He wrote an excellent article about LDN and shared the Low Dose Naltrexone website.[79] The LDN website lists the various autoimmune diseases, cancers, and other diseases that LDN helps with. This site also shared a study that showed complete remission from Crohn's disease is achievable. LDN is approved for "on-label" use for Crohn's but must be prescribed "off-label" for Hashimoto's and other autoimmune diseases. The reason for that is because there are not enough research studies for LDN as a treatment for Hashimoto's disease. Studies are costly and are often funded by drug companies with the purpose of financial gain. This drug is relatively inexpensive so there is not a lot to gain. Sadly, the potential for helping people with autoimmune thyroid conditions is not enough of a reason to fund a research study. On the positive side, there is an abundance of clinical data from doctors, pharmacists, and practitioners that have been using LDN for their Hashimoto's patients.

Some people go into complete remission by using LDN. Some patients with **thyroid antibodies over 1000 IU/mL reduced their antibodies to less than 100 IU/mL with LDN**. Many people have been able to reduce or eliminate their symptoms and reduce or stop taking thyroid hormone medications. LDN is recommended to people with high antibodies, people with multiple autoimmune conditions, and to women that want to get pregnant. LDN can also be used as an alternative treatment for Graves' disease.

While researching for this book, I was so pleased to find many newer resources on LDN, including the LDN Research Trust[80] and LDNscience.[81] Both websites assist patients with finding a prescriber. There are also several independent sites for doctors that prescribe LDN. Back in 2014, it was a little challenging to find a prescriber. I had learned that some neurologists prescribe it for Multiple Sclerosis and after getting a "no" from my primary physician, I got my first LDN prescription from a neurologist that was located one hour away. It should not be difficult to find a physician that is willing to prescribe this medication. Doctors should be more knowledgeable about autoimmune disease and should be more than willing to prescribe a medication that helps.

I suggest that you ask your doctor for this medication if you have autoimmune disease. You might get a no simply because it is still "off-label" for Hashimoto's. Don't give up. That is not a valid reason to be denied a medication that can help your condition without hurting you. If you share the resources above with your doctor, that should help. If not, you can find a prescriber online. Once prescribed, you can order LDN from a compounding pharmacy and have it mailed to your home. I recommend the Care First Specialty Pharmacy.

Remission

Although many doctors say there is no cure for Hashimoto's and do not treat it, remission is attainable! I am happy to say I am currently in remission. My TSH, Free T3, and Free T4 are all within the normal range. My TPO antibodies are also in normal range. I do not currently take thyroid medication. I do take LDN. I have reached remission several times, but Hashimoto's is like a roller coaster. We all have triggers that can push us out of balance.

In January of 2023, I recovered from several stressful events to my mind and body, including Covid-19, followed by a gallbladder attack a few weeks later. I conquered those problems with various techniques including diet, nutraceuticals, and frequency healing.

While my lab work indicates that I am currently in remission, I know I might not stay there. However, I have the tools and the knowledge to rebalance myself and feel better. That is empowering!

Our bodies have tremendous healing abilities.

CHAPTER 8

Detoxify Heavy Metals

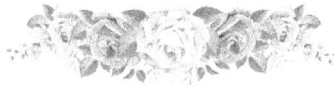

"The body is your temple. Keep it pure and clean for the soul to reside in."
– B.K.S. Iyengar

Heavy metals toxicity is a serious problem and should never be ignored. Ironically, most mainstream medical doctors never even raise the subject. Heavy metals (and other toxins) are one of the most common and overlooked causes of unexplained health problems. If you have brain fog, mood swings, fatigue, or other symptoms that your doctor hasn't helped you with, there's a good chance toxicity is the root cause.

I asked several physicians to test me for heavy metals over the years. A couple of them would not run the testing. Two mainstream doctors ordered blood tests. I visited an integrative doctor, and he ordered a six-hour urine challenge test. The urine challenge is considered the most accurate test for *long-term* exposure to most heavy metals.

In Chapter 6, you learned about the health problems associated with heavy metals, including autoimmune disease. In this chapter, you will learn about heavy metals testing and detoxification methods.

How to Avoid Exposure to Heavy Metals

Detoxifying heavy metals and other toxins is essential to healing. It removes the burden that is preventing your body from achieving healing and balance. It's important to assess which metals and toxins you have been exposed to and take action to avoid those exposures.

- Only drink clean water. Invest in a whole-house water filtration system, or at least a high-quality water filter for your drinking and bathing water. Municipal tap water is a significant source of toxins. Activated carbon filters are considered superior and remove the most contaminants, including heavy metals and pesticides. High-quality activated carbon filters can even remove pharmaceutical residues. Reverse-osmosis filters have been shown to effectively remove perchlorate, pesticides, PCBs, plastics, chloride, and a wide variety of heavy metals. Water pitcher filters do not filter out as many toxins. However, water pitcher filters using activated carbon, ion exchange resins, or nanofiltration, remove heavy metals (including arsenic, lead, chromium, nickel, and copper).
- Eat organic food as much as possible to avoid excessive pesticides and herbicides. Do not use chemicals on your lawn or garden.
- Ensure you have optimal levels of iodine and selenium. Optimal iodine and selenium intake has been found

to lessen the toxic effects that heavy metals and perchlorate can have on the thyroid.

- Do not allow your dentist to use amalgam fillings. If you have amalgam fillings, consider having them removed and do a mercury detox during the process.
- Do not use mercury-containing thermometers or light bulbs. If one breaks, make sure you follow the correct procedures to clean up the spill and dispose of the mercury.[82]
- Do not use synthetic antibacterial products, such as hand sanitizers, antibacterial cleaning products and antibacterial wipes.
- Do not use deodorant with aluminum, and avoid the use of baking soda, antacids, and other products that contain a lot of aluminum.
- Try to limit the use of plastics at home. If you use plastic products, look for "BPA-free" options. However, keep in mind that BPA-free products may still contain other bisphenol derivatives with potential thyroid-disrupting effects, so it really may be best to entirely avoid drinking from or storing food in plastic containers.
- Stop using non-stick cookware. PFOA from non-stick cookware can leach into food and is subsequently ingested. Use stainless steel, glass, or enameled cast iron cookware instead.
- Be very cautious regarding vaccinations because they contain adjuvants, such as formaldehyde and aluminum, which are used to create an inflammatory response. Aluminum has the unique ability to pass through the blood brain barrier and has been shown to have serious neurologic and psychiatric side effects.[83] Adjuvants can cause an abnormal immune inflammatory reaction, which has been shown to bring on autoimmune disease.[84] Your doctor should be aware that thyroiditis and other thyroid disorders can be induced by various

adjuvants in vaccines. You should not be given any non-essential vaccinations, especially if you are genetically predisposed to autoimmune diseases.

- Beware of silicone implants. Cases of Hashimoto's thyroiditis and subacute thyroiditis (a rare type of thyroiditis that causes pain and discomfort in the thyroid) were observed after exposure to vaccines and after exposure to silicone implantation.[85]

Testing for Heavy Metals

It may not be apparent if you have a toxic buildup of heavy metals in the body. Toxic heavy metals can be stored for many years in the tissues of the body such as bone, red blood cells, fat, nerves, brain, liver, and kidneys. Thus, it is very important to be tested for heavy metals to determine if this is challenging your health. Heavy metals are a known causative factor for autoimmune disease.

Unfortunately, heavy metals testing isn't as straightforward as you might expect it to be. There are several different tests that can be ordered by physicians. Heavy metals can be tested by examining the blood, urine, hair, and even the fingernails or toenails.

Some tests measure recent exposure to certain heavy metals while others can assess long-term exposure. If heavy metals have accumulated in your body over the course of many years, they need some help to be released and detoxed. For example, you may have heard that Alzheimer's patients sometimes have a high level of aluminum in their brains when autopsied. This demonstrates that metals accumulate in the brain.

Although there is some dissention among health experts, a urine challenge test seems to be the most effective test to determine if you have accumulated heavy metals. It is sometimes passed on because it requires you to have a chelation drug administered.

The following overview of testing methods shows that each test has its pros and cons. Keep in mind when choosing your testing method that you may have long-term exposures from childhood or young adulthood. For example, you may have had long-term exposure if you were a smoker, if you had dental amalgams, or if you lived in a polluted area or an area near industrial sites.

Simple Urine Test

A simple urine test gives an accurate indication of recent exposure of some metals. However, if there has been no recent exposure, it can give you a very low or negative result, even though you might have heavy metals you were exposed to in the past. Some heavy metals are more easily excreted from the kidneys than others. Lead and *methyl* mercury are bound to protein structures in the body and do not show up in urine tests.

A simple urine test can provide accurate results ONLY for the following heavy metals:

- **Cadmium**: Cadmium is concentrated in the kidneys, so the cadmium urine test result indicates your cumulative cadmium exposure over the long term.
- **Arsenic**: Urine is the best test for *recent* arsenic exposure only because 80 percent is excreted in urine after three days.
- **Mercury**: Urine is the best indicator of *inorganic* and *elemental* mercury exposure and kidney burden.

Urine Challenge Test

The urine challenge test is considered by many as the most accurate test for most heavy metals. If your doctor orders this test, you are given a chelating agent such as DMPA, DMSA or EDTA orally or by I.V. For the next six hours, you collect your urine in a receptable they provide. Then you collect a small sample, and mail it to the lab.

The chelating agent helps the body release heavy metals that may be lodged in your organs such as your liver, kidneys, or brain. The chelation drug essentially starts to chelate out the metals or shake things up so that metals start to be released. Those metals then start circulating around the body which can cause some unpleasant detox symptoms. That is why doctors doing this procedure should also give you glutathione. When you are given glutathione (the body's master antioxidant), the detox symptoms are minimal or nonexistent.

Whole Blood Test

This test examines the heavy metal concentrations inside your red and white blood cells The level of heavy metals found only show your exposure over the last 120 days. The heavy metals that have an affinity with red blood cells are:

- **Lead**: Whole blood is the best indicator of lead status. Around 95 percent of lead is bound to red blood cells, while the rest binds to bone and other protein structures.
- **Mercury**: Whole blood is the best indicator of organic (methyl or ethyl) mercury exposure with 70–95 percent bound to hemoglobin in red blood cells. However, blood is not an accurate indicator of inorganic or elemental mercury levels.
- **Cadmium**: Whole blood cadmium levels reflect recent exposure within the last 50 days, but not overall or long-term toxicity levels.

Blood Plasma Test

This test examines the heavy metals in the fluid surrounding our red and white blood cells. The main reason to order this test is if there is liver or kidney damage. It will only show recent exposure or severe toxicity. Blood plasma testing does not show stored metals in the body or long-term exposure unless the tissue is saturated and toxicity levels are very high.

Hair Mineral Test

A hair mineral analysis is the fastest and most affordable way to find out if you have mineral deficiencies and heavy metal toxicity. Your report will show a range for each heavy metal so you can assess how toxic you are with each metal. The minerals section of the report shows if you are deficient or if you have too much of a certain mineral which can also be a problem. You can go to a health practitioner, or you can order a hair mineral test online.

Takeaway

The doctor that you choose to request heavy metals testing from will have their own idea of what tests to run. They may not differentiate between short-term and long-term exposure, but you can use the information in this chapter to have an informed discussion and decide on the appropriate tests for you.

Preparing to Detox

If you read about every new detox program that comes out, you can become utterly confused and throw your hands up. Take it from someone who has tried many detoxes! I've attended entire detox summits with the experts discussing their programs in detail. I've also worked with other health coaches, and I have various detox programs including hundreds of recipe books at my disposal. Despite having so many choices, I have discovered a few key products that are proven to be effective, and that I recommend without hesitation. They are described in this chapter.

During the week before you start to detox, increase your hydration, exercise daily, and start transitioning to the detox diet described in this chapter. You must also make sure you are not constipated.

The pathways by which the metals leave the body need to be clear and flowing so that the metals do not recirculate in the body and cause discomfort. Ideally, twice daily you should be having a smooth, easy bowel movement, solid, soft, and well-formed (like a banana).

Otherwise, the metals that are released from your tissues might recirculate through your body, causing detox symptoms. Typical detox symptoms include diarrhea, body aches, headaches, fatigue, skin eruptions, and mood swings, however, there are ways to minimize these issues.

Warning—Do not detox if you are chronically constipated

The causes of constipation include hypothyroidism, infections, magnesium deficiency, probiotic imbalance, food allergies, dehydration, lack of exercise, or poor diet. If you have been having issues with constipation, you can try home remedies for constipation, hydrating, and eating more fiber. You can also try an enema.

You may want to consider colon therapy. Colon cleansing is where a therapist inserts a tube into your rectum, and pumps warm water in, a little at a time, massaging your abdomen to help you release the waste from your colon (the large intestine). It's also called colonic hydrotherapy or colonic irrigation. It can be used to treat constipation, or an impacted bowel and it has several potential health benefits. These include:

- Clearing waste and "toxins" from the body
- Improving digestion
- Boosting your immune function
- Aiding weight loss
- Improving mood
- Lowering colon cancer risk

I call it cleaning out the pipes! Having a colon therapist observe your stool can be awkward but it's interesting to meet someone that does this for a living. They are really into it. Why? I have no idea!

Funny story—I was talked into getting a colonic from an older friend of mine. I was only around 30 years old. So, my poo is floating along through a horizontal glass tube placed right in front of me. I'm like, "Holy shit, this is weird," and suddenly the therapist who was about 70 years old and quite stern says to me, "You have hairy balls." I quickly presumed she must have been talking crap, but I had a wisecrack! I replied, "I thought only men had those!" It took her a good five seconds to realize I was joking and then she laughed (barely). She was seriously into her shit! Turns out the hairy balls indicated that I had parasites. Ewww! I was done.

It was several years later when I decided to go for colon therapy again after suffering with chronic constipation due to a low T3 level. That's what I attributed it to. This was before being diagnosed with Hashimoto's. I had to draw my own conclusion because none of my doctors at that time were helpful.

I took Armour desiccated thyroid hormone medication for one year and I was never constipated again. My T3 level went up from being low in the range (not out of range), to middle of the range. I stopped taking the Armour after one year because my heart started beating very fast at night. I even went to a heart doctor and wore a halter to monitor my heart for 24 hours. Nothing was wrong. The Armour thyroid medication caused it. It became too much for me and I weaned myself off it. The rapid heartbeat did not return.

Foods to Eat While Detoxing Heavy Metals

Leafy green veggies: Greens are some of the best heavy metal detox foods. Try to eat some greens every day, such as spinach, kale, arugula, swiss chard, dandelion greens, mustard greens, or beet greens. Broccoli sprouts are exceptionally nutritious and therapeutic. They reduce inflammation and provide a significant amount of antioxidants. Chapter 14 provides more detail about sulforaphane, the active component of broccoli sprouts.

Foods rich in vitamin C: Fruits and vegetables rich in vitamin C help reduce the damage caused by heavy metals by acting as an antioxidant. High vitamin C foods include citrus fruits like oranges or grapefruit, leafy greens like spinach and kale, all kinds of berries, broccoli and cruciferous veggies, papaya, guava, kiwi, and bell pepper.

Herbs and spices: Anti-inflammatory, antioxidant herbs, and spices like basil, rosemary, thyme, parsley, oregano, ginger, cilantro, turmeric, and cinnamon can help remove heavy metals. Cilantro is a well-known chelator that can detoxify and reduce the heavy metals like mercury and lead in the body. You can drink cilantro or parsley juice shots or add the fresh juice to your fresh juice or smoothie. You might want to try the Medical Medium's recipe for a heavy metal detox smoothie.

Garlic, onions, and cruciferous vegetables: Sulfur-rich foods support glutathione production which helps your body detoxify itself of heavy metals.

Flax, pumpkin, and chia seeds: These seeds provide omega-3 fats, minerals, and fiber that can help with detoxification of the colon and reduce inflammation.

Water: Drink 8 ounces of water or vegetable juice every couple of hours to stay hydrated and help flush out the toxins.

Aloe Vera: Drink aloe vera juice to assist your body in breaking down and removing toxins.

Bone broth: Bone broth helps to keep you hydrated, contains minerals, and supports liver health by providing glutathione. It also contains amino acids that help strengthen the gut lining and organs.

Foods to Avoid While Detoxing

Fish: Farmed fish (especially fish from farms that are not carefully regulated) can contain heavy metals, PCBs, and dioxins, all of which are highly toxic. Fish to avoid include shark, king mackerel, swordfish, tilefish, and bigeye tuna. If you choose to eat fish, keep it on the low side, just a few times per week and choose wild-caught fish that are low in mercury.

Food allergens: Avoid eating foods your body is sensitive or allergic to. This causes inflammation and prevents your body from detoxifying optimally.

Alcohol: Too much alcohol is toxic to the body and makes it more difficult for your liver to detoxify other toxins.

Processed and non-organic foods: Avoid processed foods and foods high in additives, preservatives, and pesticides. These foods increase exposure to chemicals which make symptoms worse and decrease your body's ability to detoxify. The following is from the Environmental Working Group's dirty dozen list.[86] It is important to nourish our cells with the highest quality food possible with the lowest amounts of pesticides.

Dirty Dozen & Clean 15
Dirty Dozen
Apples, green beans, kale, collard and mustard greens, cherries, grapes, nectarines, peaches, bell and hot peppers, spinach, strawberries, blueberries.
Clean 15
Clean 15 Onions, avocados, sweet corn, pineapple, mangos, sweet peas, mushrooms, papaya, asparagus, kiwi, cabbage, carrots, honeydew melon, watermelon, sweet potatoes.

Chelation Therapy

Before pulling out the big guns and getting IV chelation, I recommend the safer and gentler detox methods described in this chapter. If you have seriously elevated levels of heavy metals, your doctor may think IV chelation might be the way to go, but you should examine all the options before proceeding.

Chelation therapy is used to reduce serious heavy metal exposure, such as lead, mercury, aluminum, and arsenic. Chelation therapy involves having a chelator drug, such as, EDTA, DMSA, or DMPS, injected into the body. Chelators attach to heavy metals, and they are eliminated through the urine and feces. Most people need between five and 30 chelation sessions for good results.

Although chelation therapy may be the most commonly used mainstream method for detoxifying heavy metals, its side effects include various toxicities such as hepatotoxicity (liver), neurotoxicity (nervous system), and other adverse reactions.[87] Glutathione must be administered with the chelation drug to prevent side effects.

I recommend that if you are considering an aggressive liver, kidney, or heavy metals detox, you consult with a licensed naturopath, functional medicine doctor, or integrative M.D. to guide you with a personalized protocol that's right for you. A gradual, gentler approach is safer, easier to handle, and can be even more effective. This chapter describes how to detox heavy metals without using harsh drugs or injections.

How to Manage Detox Reactions

Detoxing too quickly by using extreme methods such as water fasting, juice cleanses, rapid weight loss, intense liver cleanses, or other accelerated methods can trigger a detox crisis, which is why I prefer a gentler approach.

Using extreme methods can cause the heavy metals to be released too quickly into the bloodstream, which can overwhelm your body's natural detoxification processes. You do not want the toxic metals to recirculate through your bloodstream and get redistributed to organs in your body, such as the liver or brain. That is why I recommend using the nutraceuticals described in the next section, which absorb the toxins like a sponge. Whatever method you choose for your detox is your decision, but it's good to know what to do if you have a reaction.

If you experience a detox reaction that is mild enough that you can handle it without horrible discomfort, you should continue treatment and take as many of the following actions as possible. These actions assist your body to eliminate the toxins as quickly and as effectively as possible:

- Drink plenty of distilled or spring water. Add fresh lemon, orange, ginger, mint, or cucumber. Aim for half your weight in ounces. If you weigh 150 pounds, drink 75 ounces daily.
- Drybrush your skin before bathing.
- Take a detox bath or at least a foot soak.
- Drink fresh juices made with fruits and vegetables.
- Get plenty of sunshine if possible.
- Allow your body to rest.
- Sweat. Other than a good workout, the best way to sweat is to use a far infrared sauna.

If your reaction is too severe, cut back on your dosage or frequency of doses. This can help calm your symptoms while allowing the healing process to continue.

Naturally Detox Heavy Metals, Pesticides, and Other Toxins

You may have heard that garlic, cilantro, and chlorella can help to detoxify mercury and other heavy metals from the body. Garlic binds to mercury and helps remove it from soft tissues such as the digestive tract. Cilantro removes mercury and heavy metals, and it has compounds that may cross the blood brain barrier and help remove mercury from the brain and central nervous system. You need a good amount however to get a therapeutic effect. Chlorella is a milder detoxification aid that can help to remove mercury from soft tissues and support the body's natural detoxification systems. These foods are helpful, especially to remove recent exposures, but are **not** enough to resolve long-term widespread toxicity.

Modified citrus pectin and zeolite (clinoptilolite) powder are both effective binders for the detoxification of harmful heavy metals, pesticides, and other agricultural and environmental toxins. Activated charcoal is also an effective binder that is used to remove many toxins and impurities. However, there is not as much clinical evidence to support it's efficacy in removing heavy metals in comparison with modified citrus pectin and zeolite.

Modified Citrus Pectin

Modified citrus pectin (MCP) is made from pectin, which is found in the white pith of citrus fruit peels. It is called "modified citrus pectin" because the pectin is altered to be a smaller molecular size. The molecules of regular, unmodified pectin are far too large to enter the bloodstream and work for cellular health. However, these modified citrus pectin molecules have a precise structure that allows them to enter the blood circulation from the digestive tract and to absorb toxins in the gut and the bloodstream. MCP is clinically proven to remove heavy metals such as lead, mercury, cadmium, and arsenic from the body without removing essential minerals.

Modified citrus pectin (MCP) is one of the safest and most advanced detoxification substances you can use.

In studies that examined the effectiveness of modified citrus pectin in removing heavy metals, the results were significant. **MCP successfully aided the elimination of toxic heavy metals, including lead, mercury, arsenic, and cadmium,** from the body by chelating the metals in the bloodstream and eliminating them in the urine. MCP is a nontoxic chelating agent that has great potential. It can be used safely for long periods of time. In fact, it is considered a safe alternative for people for whom chelation drugs are contraindicated.[88]

Some chelation substances can remove beneficial minerals from the body but MCP does not. Studies have shown that when using MCP, **minerals are preserved in the body**.

Recommendations

It is recommended to start slow, and then increase your dosage so that you do not detox too quickly.

If you are taking capsules, you can start with two capsules twice daily, then four capsules twice daily, then six capsules, all the way up to nine capsules twice daily. One scoop of the powder is equal to six capsules. I find it easier to just mix a scoop into a smoothie, yogurt, or applesauce.

For serious conditions including autoimmune disease, 7.5 grams twice daily is the recommended dose. This is 1.5 scoops of the MCP powder or nine capsules.

During this detox, it is recommended to incorporate glutathione-supporting supplements, combined with liver detoxification

herbs (or a formula) that contains herbs such as milk thistle, dandelion root, burdock root, chanca piedra, ginger root, artichoke leaf extract, and beet root.

If you experience detoxification side effects such as headache, mood swings, or stomach upset, stay on the current dose for a few days until the symptoms pass and drink plenty of water, and then increase your dose. As a rule, when detoxing, you should drink water in the amount of half of your body weight in ounces. For example, if you weigh 200 pounds, drink 100 ounces of water daily.

After finishing your intensive detox, you can continue with a maintenance dose on an ongoing basis. Remember, the accumulation of heavy metals and toxins in your body has happened over a long period of time, so it will take time to clear them from the body. It could take several weeks or months depending on your level of toxicity.

Chapter 14 provides more detail about MCP, including scientific evidence for its numerous benefits.

Zeolite Powder

Zeolite is a natural mineral of volcanic origin. It results from a chemical reaction between lava and salt water. There are many types of zeolites but clinoptilolite is the form that is safe to use by humans for health purposes. Clinoptilolite has been shown to eliminate toxic heavy metals, including mercury, lead, arsenic, and cadmium as well as pesticides. It does not remove minerals and electrolytes from the body. It has been used for centuries as a safe remedy for removing heavy metals due to its filtering properties.

Studies have shown that clinoptilolite binds to and removes heavy metals such as lead, arsenic, and mercury. Zeolite is an effective remedy for smokers and people exposed to heavy metals in contaminated water, amalgam fillings, or through job-related exposure.

Recommendations

To detox, add a minimum of one tablespoon of zeolite clinoptilolite into a beverage or shake and drink it once or twice daily. A full heavy metal detox with clinoptilolite may take approximately two months, depending on your weight, age, health, lifestyle, and diet.

Zeolite has no known side effects. Normal detox side effects such as headaches and nausea can occur but it's uncommon. **Note:** You must drink plenty of water to prevent constipation.

Chapter 14 provides more detail about zeolite, including more dosing information and scientific evidence for its numerous benefits.

Vitamin E, Methyl Folate, Selenium, and Curcumin

If you have arsenic toxicity, consider taking vitamin E. Studies have shown that vitamin E helps to reduce arsenic levels. You should also be sure to get enough selenium and methyl folate, which can help your body excrete arsenic. A diet rich in selenium and other antioxidants may prevent arsenic toxicity.[89]

You may also consider taking either curcumin or tetrahydrocurcumin. Curcumin was found to repair DNA damage caused by arsenic toxicity, and thereby prevent arsenic-induced carcinogenesis.[90] A metabolite of curcumin, tetrahydrocurcumin has even more impressive benefits. See Chapter 13 for details.

Activated Charcoal

Activated charcoal has been used for decades to support natural detoxification. One of its benefits is that it it is safe to take on a daily basis. The porous structure of activated charcoal enables it to bind to and trap various toxins and impurities in the digestive system. As the charcoal moves through the gastrointestinal tract, like a sponge, it attracts and adsorbs harmful substances and prevents their absorption into the body.

Ozonated charcoal is reportedly 10 times as effective as activated charcoal, according to Dr. Edward Group of Global Healing. You will learn more about activated charcoal in Chapter 14.

Recommendations

Take activated charcoal or ozonated activated charcoal alone 60 to 90 minutes before eating or taking any other supplements or medication.

Fiber is Important While Detoxing

To avoid the side effects of detoxing, it helps to consume fiber, as it assists with absorbing toxins and transporting them out of the body. The reason many people feel awful while detoxing is because toxins are pulled out of the blood and tissues and can get recirculated throughout the body.

If you are eating a healthy whole food diet while detoxing, the fiber in your food will help to trap and absorb the toxins your liver is dumping into your GI tract. Those toxins are then transported out of your body through bowel movements.

If you are not eating any fiber because you are on a "juice fast" or a "juice cleanse" you might have a problem. Some detox programs advise you to drink only fiber-less juice such as wheatgrass juice, celery juice, carrot juice, etc., while at the same time taking strong detox supplements. However, if you don't have any fiber to trap the toxins that your liver is releasing into your small intestines, the toxins can be reabsorbed through your gastrointestinal tract.

Smooth Moves

It is important when detoxing to make sure the toxins have a pathway to leave the body without reabsorbing. Make sure your bowels are moving regularly, preferable two or three bowel movements per day. If you are not having smooth moves, you can use herbal laxative capsules or tea. I had the best results with Triple Leaf Tea and Natural Balance Colon Clenz capsules. If you suffer with constipation, you must address and resolve this problem. Eating more fiber and drinking more water is not always enough. Eliminating gluten is the solution for many people. However, if you have other reasons for your constipation, you may need some help to determine the cause. Having low thyroid hormone and eating gluten were two things that contributed to my constipation. After eliminating gluten and normalizing my T3 level, my constipation resolved.

My Personal Metals Detox Journey

I was mercury-poisoned as a young girl by my dentist. And so was everyone else back then that had multiple cavities filled with amalgams. I had eleven amalgam fillings. The mercury in those fillings continued to escape into my blood every time I ate or drank for decades. The more fillings you have, the more poison gets released into your body. Mercury is bioaccumulative, which means it accumulates in your tissues. There is NO safe level of mercury. When I was tested for mercury, I had a very high level and that led me to investigate how it happened.

History of Amalgam (Mercury) Fillings

Amalgam is an alloy that typically consists of **50 percent mercury**. It also contains silver, tin, and zinc. The following timeline of amalgam history is shocking.

- 1830s: Amalgam fillings were introduced into American dentistry.

- 1840: The American Society of Dental Surgeons were concerned about mercury poisoning and required members to **denounce** the use of amalgams. Many dentists continued using amalgams since they preferred them to gold fillings due to ease of use and price.
- 1844: 50 percent of all dental restorations reported in upstate New York were amalgam. At that time, using dental amalgam was **malpractice**.
- 1859: The dentists who continued using amalgam fillings in America formed their own dental society, the National Dental Association, which became the **American Dental Association (ADA)**. The ADA strongly fought against people claiming that dental amalgam was harmful to our health. Why did the ADA knowingly put so many people in harm's way? Because amalgam was cheap, durable, and easier to work with. Patients be damned.
- Amalgam fillings were used as the primary material for restoring teeth for over 150 years in the United States.

> **The American Dental Association (ADA) knowingly poisoned millions of people for 150 years.**

The European Commission plans to phase out dental amalgam and mercury-containing light bulbs and lamps in 2025.[91] South Africa and New Zealand are also planning to phase out amalgams. In the US, many dental schools are teaching dentists how to use composite or glass ionomer fillings which has resulted in less use of amalgam fillings.[92] There should be ZERO amalgam fillings.

Continuous Mercury Vapor Leakage

The International Academy of Oral Medicine & Toxicology asserts that mercury vapor continuously leaks from dental amalgam fillings, and a lot of it gets absorbed into the body's tissues. The level of mercury "microleakage" is associated with the number of fillings and common activities, such as chewing food, drinking hot liquids, and teeth-grinding. Mercury also gets released when filling, replacing, and removing dental amalgam fillings.[93]

Replaced All Amalgam Fillings

Before I was tested for heavy metals toxicity, I found a holistic dentist and spoke to him about having my amalgam fillings removed. After researching, I was concerned that my fillings were affecting my health and contributing to my eczema. The eczema was making me miserable. I shelled out about $2,200 to get all my fillings replaced. The dentist gave me a bottle of homeopathic drops for detoxification. I did not know much about detoxing metals at the time. I took about half of the bottle and just got on with my life. In retrospect, I think I was exposed to mercury toxicity while the fillings were being removed. I felt the crumbled bits of fillings in my mouth during the process. I wish I knew then what I know now. I would have at least taken Pectasol-C and taken clay baths to get the mercury out. Just a couple years later, my younger son was born with autism. A couple years later, I tested both of my children for mercury with a urine test at home. Only the youngest tested positive for mercury, not the eldest. This led me to believe that I may have incurred more mercury toxicity during the process of removal.

EDTA Chelation

About 10 years later, I was tested for heavy metals with two urine challenge tests using two different chelators. A chelator is a chelation drug (such as EDTA) that starts to pull the metals out from your brain and other organs. I was injected with a different chelator specifically for aluminum.

The results showed that I was high in **mercury, aluminum, lead, and arsenic.**

I received Intravenous (IV) EDTA chelation treatment every two weeks for six months. I was given glutathione each time I received the EDTA chelation therapy to support detoxification and prevent the detoxification side effects. After six months of treatments, I repeated the urine challenge. The doctor said he couldn't give me glutathione with the EDTA injection because he wanted to retest my urine. Boy did I feel the difference! I felt wretched (malaise, fatigue, pain, skin eruptions, and mood swings) after getting EDTA without the glutathione. To be fair, they said that I could go back to get the glutathione a few days later. But I figured it would go away, and it was a 45-minute drive, and I could not make it there due to my hectic schedule as a single working mom. Instead, I just waited for the results of the test anxiously. When I finally received a call, it was to tell me that the lab dropped my urine sample and spilled all of it! They said I would have to repeat the test. I was exasperated. I had just undergone two weeks of misery. I decided not to repeat that procedure or return to Dr. Jerk after the way he had treated myself and my boys for the past few months. I was done. He was firrrrredd!!!

Did EDTA chelation therapy work for me? It may have but I'll never know. I did not receive the urine test results due to the lab spilling my entire sample! Regardless, I did not notice any improvement in my symptoms after those six months of EDTA chelation. I did observe major improvements in the following year however, after using the safe and natural chelation supplements, modified citrus pectin and zeolite powder, combined with other supplements. I did courses of both of those to shrink my thyroid nodules, and they also functioned as a heavy metals cleanse!

In retrospect, I would not recommend EDTA chelation. I would like to think that it helped me, but my symptoms did not improve at that time. Recently, about 10 years later, another doctor ordered heavy metals testing on my blood (not urine). I didn't have any heavy metals out of range. That might indicate that I am no longer toxic with heavy metals, OR just that I was not recently exposed. I think it is safe to say that I have resolved or at least significantly lowered my metals toxicity. I resolved the depression, anxiety, and fatigue that I was suffering with before the heavy metals cleanse. I also achieved remission from Hashimoto's and shrunk my thyroid nodules.

Natural Heavy Metals Cleanse

The first time I did a *natural* heavy metals cleanse, the primary goal was to shrink my thyroid nodules, but this approach served multiple purposes. I took supplements that are clinically proven to detox the body of heavy metals. I took the intensive dose of the Pectasol-C brand of modified citrus pectin (5 grams, three times a day) for several weeks. Next, I took Pure brand or HealthForce Nutritionals brand zeolite (clinoptilolite) powder (1 tbsp per day) for two weeks. I then alternated back to Pectasol-C. I continued alternating for several months. I also took supplements to support glutathione production and detoxification (described below).

I felt a significant improvement afterwards. I felt lighter, happier, more energetic, and my concentration and mental clarity improved significantly.

I did not follow a liquid diet, but I did eat lighter. I eliminated gluten, dairy, eggs, grains, and all meat with the exception of a small amount of chicken in a homemade soup. I consumed more liquids, including lemon water with mint and chia seeds. I found that detoxing naturally without an extreme diet was manageable, effective, and helped me to feel better and maintain my strength. Best of all, it helped to shrink my thyroid nodules and alleviate my fear of cancer.

I continue to use Pectasol-C regularly to maintain my health and prevent cancer and toxicity.

Glutathione and Supporting Supplements

Glutathione is your body's master antioxidant and detoxifier. It kills free radicals, prevents aging, and supports skin health and immune health. It is one of the most important antioxidants for heavy metals detoxification.

The following supplements support your body's production of glutathione and help detoxify mercury and other heavy metals from the body:

- **Alpha lipoic acid** helps restore glutathione levels due to immune system depletion
- **Vitamin C** helps raise glutathione in red blood cells and lymphocytes
- **Selenium** is required for your body to make glutathione
- **N-Acetyl Cysteine (NAC)** is a natural pre-cursor to glutathione
- **Liposomal glutathione** encapsulates the glutathione molecule inside of a lipid to improve absorption

I continue to take all these supplements but usually opt for NAC instead of liposomal glutathione because it may not be as bioavailable as NAC. NAC is absorbed in the gastrointestinal tract, goes to the liver, and gets converted to cysteine, which the liver uses to produce glutathione. The recommended dose of NAC is 600–1,800 mg daily, which can be effective against many conditions.[94]

Happy Days

What I noticed after two months of alternating courses of zeolite powder and modified citrus pectin was that I was feeling lighter and happier, and I had a lot more energy! I was flying high. In fact, I was so cheerful at work, I think I was annoying some of my grouchy coworkers! The results from these nutraceuticals were clearly noticeable.

Takeaway

Whether you have heavy metals testing performed or not, most people are toxic with some degree of metals, pesticides, and other pollutants just by virtue of the toxicity that exists in our food, air, and water at this time in history. The detoxification steps described in this chapter, including the binders, supplements, dietary tips, and the importance of fiber and smooth elimination, are all important parts of eliminating toxins and helping you to heal and reverse disease.

CHAPTER 9

Eradicate Viral Cells

"Viruses don't just make us sick. They can actually sometimes end up in our genomes."
— Carl Zimmer

Reducing viral cells that remain in your body from past infections can improve your health by removing a major root cause of many diseases, including Hashimoto's. The effects of the Epstein-Barr virus in particular are serious and are becoming more understood, particularly in the alternative medicine community. The best medicine for this issue is natural medicine.

Natural Antiviral Medicine

The foods, herbs, essential oils, and nutraceuticals described in this section have been shown to reduce various types of viral cells, including (but not limited to) EBV. These items can be used in various forms, including tea, liquid extract (tincture), essential oil, capsules, or included in food or beverages. It depends on each item, your preference, and the reason for taking it. Obviously, you don't have to take all these items at the same time. You can alternate and do courses of various supplements while including the fresh herbs in your diet.

Antiviral Nutraceuticals

Some of the top nutraceuticals that fight viruses include Vitamin C, L-lysine, lemon balm, cat's claw (Uña de gato), oregano oil, zinc, N-Acetyl Cysteine (NAC), astragalus, echinacea, beta glucans, holy basil, olive leaf extract, berberine, and licorice root.

Berberine: Berberine is an herb known for lowering glucose but it also has antiviral, anticancer, and anti-inflammatory properties. Berberine has been shown in studies to target EBV and several other herpes viruses, including HSV-1, HSV-2, and cytomegalovirus virus.[95]

Elderberry: Elderberry is a strong antiviral and supports the immune system.

L-lysine: L-lysine is an essential amino acid that helps to fight all herpes family viruses, including EBV. It impairs the ability of viral cells to move and reproduce. L-lysine is a powerful agent in the fight against cancer, liver disease, inflammation, atherosclerosis, and the symptoms and conditions caused by viruses.

Red clover: Red clover can help cleanse the liver, spleen, and lymphatic system of neurotoxins left by the EBV virus.

Reishi (Lingzhi) Mushroom: Reishi mushroom, also known as Lingzhi, is rich in beta glucans. It is one of the best, if not THE best plant in the world for finding, decomposing, and flushing out cellular waste from your body. This allows the surrounding blood vessels and organs to function more efficiently. Reishi is loaded with terpenes. It makes sense that one of its innate abilities is to do a similar breaking-down and dissipating action in the body.

Uña de gato: Uña de gato, also known as cat's claw, is one of the most powerful tools in fighting EBV, shingles, and other herpes viruses. It is also used to fight bacterial and parasitic infections.

Zinc: Ionic zinc fights viruses in multiple ways. It also strengthens the immune system against EBV.

Antiviral Foods and Herbs

Some of the top foods and herbs that fight viruses include garlic, ginger, basil, oregano, green tea, and turmeric.

The following foods are known to specifically fight EBV and support thyroid health:

Wild Blueberries: Wild blueberries are smaller than the larger commonly grown varieties. They can be found in the freezer section of many supermarkets. They are also available in a concentrated powder form. Wild blueberries help to flush EBV neurotoxins out of the liver which helps the nervous system. They also bind to and help remove toxic heavy metals from the brain and liver. They contain powerful antioxidants that help repair your thyroid gland and reduce the growth of nodules.

Apples: Apples reduce inflammation in the thyroid because the apple pectin enters the digestive system and releases phytochemicals that bind to EBV and prevent the viral cells from growing.

Avocados: Avocados contain a form of copper that helps to balance T3 and T4 production.

Bananas: Bananas have powerful antiviral and anti-inflammatory properties. Bananas provide amino acids and a type of potassium that helps to rebuild EBV-damaged neurotransmitters. They are a great source of calcium because banana trees grow in calcium-rich soil. There is no need to worry about their sugar content (as some warn) because they actually help to balance blood sugar. Their fruit sugar serves as high-quality brain food and it bonds to its amino acids and minerals, making it an awesome superfood.

Basil: Basil is antiviral. It has phytochemical compounds that go into the thyroid and slow down EBV activity. Basil also fights cancer. It helps reduce nodules, cysts, and tumors and it has anticancer compounds that help prevent thyroid cancer.

Berries: Berries are highly beneficial to the thyroid. They are high in antioxidants and help to prevent thyroid tissue damage. Blackberries help slow the growth of nodules and strengthen thyroid tissue. Raspberries bind to and remove EBV, viral debris, and other impurities from the bloodstream.

Cilantro: Cilantro binds to EBV neurotoxins and to toxic heavy metals like mercury (which feed the EBV virus).

Coconut: Coconut is antiviral and anti-inflammatory. It kills EBV cells and prevents nodule growth. It also helps prevents nervous system imbalance caused by EBV neurotoxins.

Garlic: Garlic is antiviral and antibacterial. It kills viral cells, including EBV and strep.

Ginger: Ginger is a powerful antiviral against EBV. Ginger helps to balance thyroid health by giving it a boost if it's hypo and calming it down if it's hyper.

Hemp seeds: Hemp seeds provide micronutrients and vital amino acids for your thyroid. They help protect the heart from EBV biofilm byproducts that can gum up valves in the heart and create heart palpitations. Hemp fortifies the cardiovascular system and helps protect other parts of the body that EBV damages, such as the eyes. For example, they can help to heal eye floaters.

Lemon and lime: Lemons and limes improve digestion by raising levels of hydrochloric acid, which is a helpful type of acid that you need to digest meals. They also help to cleanse the liver and balance calcium and sodium levels in the blood, improving electrolyte balance, which can improve brain fog and other neurological symptoms caused by EBV neurotoxins.

Lettuce: Lettuce (especially butter, leaf, and romaine lettuce) stimulates peristaltic action in the intestinal tract and helps cleanse EBV from the liver and lymphatic system. Lettuce is a blood cleanser. It contains trace mineral salts that support the adrenal glands, which ends up helping thyroid health.

Mango: Mangoes have plenty of carotene which nourishes the spleen and liver, feeds the brain, and helps the lymphatic system let go of EBV toxins.

Antiviral Essential Oils

I earned a certificate in aromatherapy as an adjunct to my health coach certification. I am not a clinically certified aromatherapist, however, I use essential oils for many purposes, and I make a lot of essential oils blends and remedies. Virtually all essential oils have multiple purposes and will benefit you in many ways when you diffuse or apply them.

Essential oils that have antiviral properties include holy basil, grapefruit, rosemary, peppermint, fennel, cinnamon, oregano, ginger, manuka, thyme, tea tree, and sage.

I recommend that you use essential oils **topically** or with a **diffuser**. You can put 100 percent pure essential oils in an aromatherapy diffuser. When you inhale the mist through your nose or mouth, airborne molecules are carried to your lungs and your respiratory system, some of which enter the bloodstream via the blood circulating in the lungs. They also reach areas in the brain's limbic system.

Note: Essential oils must be diluted before you apply them to your skin. You should use a prepared blend or add a few drops of a pure essential oil to a quality carrier oil, such as coconut oil, golden jojoba oil, or avocado oil.

Warning: Oral ingestion (swallowing) of essential oils is NOT recommended because there are multiple risks including burning the mucosal membranes, toxicity to the liver and kidneys, interactions with other medications, and chemical breakdown during digestion that can change the effects. Significant essential oils knowledge and expertise is needed for safe practice. Although some essential oils can be used internally, they are very strong. Some people take them in capsules. I personally do not take them internally as medicine, but I do occasionally use a few drops when cooking to flavor certain recipes. If you want to take any of them internally, you should work with a qualified aromatherapist, herbalist, or doctor. Keep in mind that if the essential oil label does not state a dosage, then it should not be taken internally.

Sample Antiviral Protocol

In my case, after learning about EBV's correlation with thyroid disease, I set out on a mission to reduce viral cells. I took a subset of the items listed above for about a month and felt a significant boost in my health. My antiviral protocol included:

- Vitamin C capsules
- L-lysine capsules
- Lemon balm liquid extract
- Ginger capsules
- Cat's claw capsules
- N-acetylcysteine (NAC) capsules
- Red clover capsules

Fresh Juices

Drinking fresh juices on an empty stomach is a great way to help your body detox while adding healthy minerals and nutrients into your bloodstream. The following are three excellent choices, especially while detoxing or treating illness.

Fresh Celery Juice

You may have heard about the celery juice craze. It's quite popular because many people all over the world are experiencing significant health improvements from a variety of conditions. Celery has special mineral salts, called sodium cluster salts. These salts are suspended in living water inside the celery plant. They are not the same as table salt, or even healthy versions of salt such as Celtic Sea salt or Himalayan salt. People on low-sodium diets can safely drink celery juice. In fact, drinking celery juice helps to remove old crystallized toxic salts from your body.

These sodium cluster salts contain trace minerals which serve many different purposes. They neutralize toxins, including copper, mercury, and aluminum, as they float through the organs of the body. They also fight harmful bacteria and viruses, including Epstein-Barr and strep. They help the liver to produce and strengthen bile, and to rejuvenate. They also help your mood by enhancing the production and quality of your neurotransmitters.

Specific benefits of fresh celery juice for people with Hashimoto's disease are:

- Fights Epstein-Barr virus
- Cleanses thyroid of viral byproducts
- Boosts production of T3
- Fights autoimmune disease
- Helps heal the gut
- Reduces inflammation

These benefits apply specifically to fresh, juiced, celery (using a juicer). Eating it or taking powdered celery pills does not have even close to the same benefits.

Twelve to 32 ounces of fresh celery juice on an empty stomach is recommended daily. Wait at least 15 to 30 minutes before eating anything.

If you cannot access celery or have an allergy to it, a healthy alternative is cucumber juice. It is not an equal substitute, but it has many benefits (described below). I personally have an allergy to celery. I have severe itching when consuming even a small amount of celery, so I drink cucumber juice instead.

Fresh Cucumber Juice

Fresh cucumber juice is an exceptionally healthy tonic for your body. It is a superior way to hydrate the body because it has electrolytes that help to bring nutrients and hydration deep into the cells and tissues. It helps to cleanse the body and release toxins. It is one of the best diuretics available, helping with the elimination of wastes through the kidneys and helping to dissolve uric acid accumulations which lead to kidney and bladder stones. It also helps reduce edema and bloating. It is alkalizing which means it reduces acidity, which helps to alleviate digestive problems such as gastritis, acidity, heartburn, indigestion, and ulcers. It is rich in nutrients including vitamins A, C, K, magnesium, silicon, and potassium.

Cucumber juice is highly anti-inflammatory and can help with autoimmune and neurological disorders such as Hashimoto's, chronic fatigue syndrome, migraines, eczema, psoriasis, rheumatoid arthritis, fibromyalgia, multiple sclerosis, and lupus. Cucumber juice is cooling and serves as an excellent aid to reduce a fever.

Twelve to 32 ounces of fresh cucumber juice (using a juicer) on an empty stomach is recommended daily. Wait at least 15 to 30 minutes before eating anything.

Aloe Vera Juice

Aloe vera is a tonic for the entire digestive system. It helps to relieve constipation, indigestion, irritable bowel syndrome (IBS), and many other digestive problems. Aloe vera also helps boost the immune system and improve skin health and dental health. Aloe vera's polysaccharide molecules help flush waste, mucus, and toxins, including pesticides and heavy metals out of the bloodstream and liver. It also supports the adrenal glands and helps to draw radiation out of the thyroid.

Aloe juice is best when made fresh from an aloe leaf. Cut a two-inch piece from a large store-bought aloe leaf, or the equivalent of smaller aloe leaves if you have a plant at home. Remove the gel and place in a blender with 16 ounces of water. Drink immediately on an empty stomach.

Recommendations

Take steps to maintain a low viral count. After you follow an antiviral regime for a few weeks or a month, you may notice an improvement in how you feel. I personally felt a noticeable difference and I hope you do too. I recommend using several of the antiviral items described in this chapter as part of your lifestyle to stay healthy.

CHAPTER 10

Essential Steps to Heal Your Gut

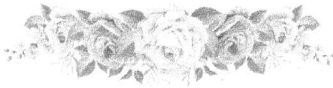

"All disease begins in the gut."
— Hippocrates

Poor gut health is one of the root causes of Hashimoto's disease. As mentioned before, there are three issues that must exist for an autoimmune disease to develop:

- Genetic predisposition
- A trigger (such as environmental toxicity or infections)
- Intestinal permeability (leaky gut)

Healing your gut is critical to improving your health if you have Hashimoto's or any autoimmune disease. It's incredible how many bodily functions are performed in our guts. Three of the major roles that gut health plays are immune regulation, mood regulation, and skin health.

Leaky Gut Syndrome

Approximately 80 percent of your immune system activity happens in your digestive tract. Your intestinal lining is naturally a little permeable so that nutrients from what you eat and drink can enter your bloodstream. However, certain foods and chemicals can damage the intestinal walls, causing increased intestinal permeability. This allows bigger food particles to seep through, as well as toxins, bacteria, and viruses. The immune system doesn't recognize these substances and does what it's designed to do. It jumps into action to fight these "invaders" which causes an inflammatory response. This inflammation becomes chronic with continuous exposure. Leaky gut can be worsened by antibiotics, candida overgrowth, stress, gut infections, and birth control pills, patches, or rings.

Some of these "foreign invaders" floating in your bloodstream look very similar to your own body's cells. Your immune system can get confused and accidentally attack your own tissues. This is called "molecular mimicry." Gluten's chemical structure is very similar to that of your thyroid tissue. So once gluten has led to leaky gut and is floating freely throughout your bloodstream, it can trigger attacks on your thyroid.

Gluten Triggers Leaky Gut

Gluten is one of the major causes of leaky gut. Gluten is a protein found in wheat, barley, and rye. It triggers the release of zonulin (a protein) in some people. Alessio Fasano M.D. is one of the leading gluten sensitivity researchers in the world. He's a gastroenterologist at Massachusetts General Hospital in Boston and head of research at the University of Harvard Celiac Research

Center. According to Dr. Fasano, "No human being completely digests gluten, and in a small percentage of us, that undigested gluten triggers the release of zonulin." Zonulin is a protein that directly causes leaky gut. High levels of zonulin cause the tight junctions in the wall of the intestine to break. This can result in symptoms resembling irritable bowel syndrome (IBS) such as bloating, abdominal pain, cramps, constipation or diarrhea, fatigue, headache, brain fog, and joint or muscle pain.[96]

In 2011, Dr. Fasano published a paper titled "Leaky Gut and Autoimmune Diseases" which introduced a new theory suggesting that prevention and reversal of autoimmune disease is possible.[97] Dr. Fasano stated that the autoimmune process can be stopped and even reversed by removing environmental and genetic triggers and by healing leaky gut.

This was a huge advancement and the first theory to present the possibility for autoimmune reversal. Research and treatment have advanced tremendously since then. Fasano showed that the damage to the gut and immune system can be modulated or reversed by **removing environmental triggers and foods with gluten**.

Another big advancement came in 2014 when Italian researchers successfully used the probiotic Lactobacillus rhamnosus GG (LGG) to prevent gliadin (gluten) from weakening the intestinal barrier. They administered gliadin which caused a release of zonulin and resulted in an increased cellular permeability in the intestinal lining. Then they administered the LGG probiotic and **the intestinal barrier was significantly restored**.[98]

GMO Foods and Glyphosate

Genetically modified organisms (GMOs) are linked to autoimmunity and other serious health problems. They contain higher amounts of pesticides and thus contribute to leaky gut.

There are approximately 61 countries (including most of the European nations, Brazil, and even China) that require labels on GMO products, but the U.S. had no such protection in place for its citizens until recently. According to the FDA, a standard was recently implemented to require labeling of bioengineered foods.[99] As of 2022, bioengineered foods sold in the United States must display information on their food packaging using one of several approved methods.[100] An estimated 75 percent of *processed* foods in U.S. stores contain GMO ingredients.[101]

There are two types of genetically modified (GM) crops:

1. Herbicide tolerant. This type of GMO crop is designed to survive high doses of toxic weed killers. The crops are heavily sprayed. These toxic weed-killing herbicides are linked to health disorders such as cancer, birth defects, hormone disruption, and autoimmune disease.

2. BT-Toxin (self-generating insecticide). Corn and cotton crops are engineered with BT-toxin. "Toxin" is in the name. BT-toxin breaks open the stomachs of insects to kill them. The stomach of the insect bursts. It has been reported that BT-toxin can also break the wall of human cells which damages the intestines and causes leaky gut.[102]

Ironically, a journal about "insect science" claims that foods with BT-toxin are not harmful to humans. Does anyone see through these claims? Do you have to immediately drop dead or get seriously ill for the harmful effects to be acknowledged? Studies have shown damage to the digestive tract. BT-toxin is designed to produce its own insecticide in each and every cell.

It's important for people with autoimmune disease to have a healthy biome, meaning plenty of beneficial bacteria. Beneficial gut bacteria help fight harmful bacteria like E. coli, botulism, and salmonella. The herbicide glyphosate, however, is a strong antibiotic that destroys our good bacteria. The damage to the biome puts people at risk for developing inflammation, candida overgrowth, and leaky gut because bad bacteria is resistant to glyphosate, and it multiplies out of control.

Inflammatory bowel disease (IBD) includes two chronic inflammatory diseases: Crohn's disease (CD) and ulcerative colitis (UC). These diseases have become prevalent all over the world. Could it be because we are being slowly poisoned by crops and processed foods with high amounts of harmful herbicides?

GMO Foods

Besides avoiding processed foods, the following are crops and products that are commonly GMO. You can avoid them by buying organic, from local farms, or growing your own.

GMO Foods		
Corn	Canola	Soy
Russet Potatoes	Yellow squash	Cottonseed
Sugar beets	Zucchini	Alfalfa
Ingredients that come from corn such as corn meal, corn gluten, corn masa, cornstarch, corn syrup, and high fructose corn syrup		
Vegetable oils and margarines made with corn, soy, cottonseed, or canola		
Ingredients that come from soybeans such as tofu, tamari, tempeh, soy protein, soy isolates, soy isoflavones, soy lecithin, soy flour, and soy protein supplements.		

National and state organic certification rules do not allow GMOs to be labeled "organic." When you buy organic, you buy food that is free not only of pesticides, but also genetically modified ingredients. The following are global standard PLU codes that help you determine if produce is conventional, organic, or GMO:

Conventional: 4-digit code starting with 4

Organic: 5-digit code starting with 9

GMO: 5-digit code starting with 8

To keep up with developments regarding the safety of our food and other products, and/or to get involved, follow the Environmental Working Group.[103]

Six Steps to Heal Your Gut

The following six steps are necessary to heal your gut. These steps can overlap and do not have to be done sequentially. For example, you can remove gluten and optimize your diet while you are doing a parasite cleanse.

1. Treat Infections and Parasites

There are several ways viral and bacterial infections may trigger Hashimoto's. I explained earlier how a leaky gut can lead to molecular mimicry, where your immune system attacks your thyroid in a case of mistaken identity. Infections can have the same effect. Your immune system mistakes your thyroid tissues for viral or bacterial cells and begins attacking.[104]

Another scenario is if the infection invades your thyroid gland or hides in its cells. When this happens, your immune system tries to kill the viral or bacterial cells and damages your thyroid as a result. Infections commonly found in people with Hashimoto's include herpes viruses, Epstein-Barr, Lyme disease, hepatitis C, H. pylori, and yersinia enterocolitica. These infections often show no symptoms, so you may not be aware that you have been infected. You should work with your medical team to eradicate any infections and then retest to check your results.

Remember, you can eliminate viral cells with natural antiviral medicines as explained in Chapter 9. You will learn how to address parasite infections later in this chapter.

2. Remove Gluten and Inflammatory Foods

Gluten triggers leaky gut. It has been proven in studies across the globe. If you have leaky gut, gluten makes it worse. You should remove it from your diet at least until your gut heals. Any other foods that inflame your gut should also be avoided until your gut heals. Refer to Chapter 11 to learn about foods that are inflammatory and foods that support the thyroid.

3. Detoxify to Remove Harmful Heavy Metals, Pesticides, and Other Toxins

We are exposed to hundreds if not thousands of toxins every day. Toxins can accumulate in your body and damage your health, including how your thyroid functions.

Many toxins cause damage to the thyroid and immune system. They include:

- **Heavy metals** such as lead, mercury, aluminum, cadmium, and arsenic
- **Perchlorates**, which interfere with the uptake of iodine by the thyroid, which can decrease thyroid hormone production
- **Halogens,** which are absorbed by your thyroid instead of iodine when you are exposed to chlorine, fluoride, and bromide. This can prevent your thyroid from having enough iodine to produce adequate levels of thyroid hormones.
- **Nitrates** are linked to increased rates of thyroid cancer. Nitrates interfere with the uptake of iodine by the thyroid, which can decrease T3 and T4 levels.[105]

- **Pesticides, herbicides, and fungicides**, which damage the intestinal lining and increase the risk of cancer and other diseases.

What to do

First assess what you are being exposed to, then look for ways to prevent your exposure to them. Many of these toxins can be in your tap water. Mercury can be found in the air (from coal burning plants), as well as in pesticides, dental fillings, fish, cosmetics, and vaccines. Lead is in the air from airplane emissions, and is also found in food, water, cosmetics, plastics, toys, and lead paint which is still used in China. In fact, more than half of paints tested in China exceeded the allowed levels.[106] Heavy metals are also found in cigarette smoke, hookah smoke, e-cigarette smoke, smokeless tobacco, marijuana, cigars, and vapes. Refer to the Heavy Metals section of Chapter 6 for more ways to avoid exposure to heavy metals.

You can remove toxins from your body with a variety of detox methods and learn ways to help your body's detoxification pathways to function optimally. The tips below will help you to minimize continued exposure:

- Filter your water in your home and shower
- Drink filtered or spring water. You can look for a local spring at the findaspring.com website, which maps springs all over the world.
- Grow or buy organic and local food
- Clean produce with veggie wash or ozonated water
- Limit consumption of large fish
- Buy pure and natural, non-toxic body products or make your own
- Have a holistic dentist safely remove amalgam fillings
- Refuse any fluoride treatments offered by dentists
- Avoid any kind of smoking
- Make informed decisions about vaccines and medications

- Use air cleaners and open windows on clear days to let fresh air flow

Glyphosate can be removed from the body with binders such as modified citrus pectin and zeolite, with the addition of N-Acetyl Cysteine (NAC), kelp, and fulvic acid. Refer to Chapter 8 for a detox strategy.

4. Replenish Your Microbiome with Healthy Bacteria and Enzymes

Many people with Hashimoto's and hypothyroidism are deficient in hydrochloric acid and digestive enzymes. This results in low levels of stomach acid, and sometimes none at all. This makes your body work much harder to digest your food and can result in poor nutrient absorption and fatigue. To replenish your biome:

- Eat fermented foods
- Take a highly rated probiotic to replenish your gut with beneficial bacteria
- Take a quality enzyme formula with meals, preferably one with betaine and pepsin. Betaine HCL and pepsin help break down proteins and make nutrients and amino acids more bioavailable.

5. Repair the Gut with Nutrients and Amino Acids

It is necessary to take quality supplements to provide your body with the nutrients it needs to conquer Hashimoto's. Some people think you can get all your nutrients from your food, but this just isn't true. Even if you eat an excellent nutritional diet, there are several reasons why that is not enough to prevent disease. Soil is often depleted, and the food grown in it does not have the expected levels of nutrients. In addition, nutrient absorption is not optimal in people with Hashimoto's. Supplements can correct nutrient deficiencies and prevent future illness. Some nutrients in large doses act as effective natural medicine, so supplementing with them can be highly beneficial to your health and longevity.

Improve Nutrient Absorption with Gut-Healing Protocols

An estimated 70-80% of our immune cells are located in our gut, so taking care of our digestive system helps our immune system. Gut healing protocols commonly include the following:

- Probiotics—Helps with immune and gastrointestinal health
- Enzymes—Help break down proteins and carbohydrates, which can reduce intestinal inflammation
- Fulvic acid—Nourishes the digestive tract and helps the good bacteria to repopulate and create a healthy microbiome.
- Biocidin—Clears irritants, unwanted microbes, and biofilms, while enhancing beneficial organisms
- Shilajit—Powerful anti-inflammatory with gut healing properties
- Aloe vera—Improves digestion and helps release clogged areas in intestines which improves the absorption of nutrients and the transport of nutrients to other areas
- Deglycyrrhized (DGL) licorice—Helps with leaky gut, ulcers, indigestion, and nausea
- Reishi mushroom—Helps modulate your immune system
- L-glutamine—Helps to repair leaky gut
- Zinc—Helps repair the intestinal barrier and tighten leaky gut
- Omega-3 fatty acids—Reduces inflammation and supports gut health
- Vitamin D—Helps immune function and gut function
- N-Acetyl-L-Cysteine (NAC)—Helps with leaky gut and protects the liver from toxins

There are many gut-repair supplements available for gut healing. Some additional gut-healing ingredients not listed above include slippery elm bark, turmeric, ginger, and marshmallow root. If a formula contains senna or cascara sagrada, take caution as these are laxatives and should not be taken on a daily basis.

Do not miss Chapter 13 where you will learn about many wonderful nutraceuticals.

Protein and Amino Acids

Eating protein-rich foods provides us with amino acids. If you don't get enough protein in your diet, you can become deficient in amino acids and other nutrients such as vitamin B12, selenium, and zinc. There are 20 amino acids that are necessary for human health. Eight are considered essential and cannot be made by your body.

Amino acids have important functions in the body and play a key role in the health of people with thyroid conditions. In fact, a deficiency can contribute to many Hashimoto's and hypothyroidism symptoms, including anxiety, muscle weakness, hair loss, poor liver health, and digestive issues. L-Tyrosine is an amino acid that is used to make thyroid hormones and glutamine, which helps to repair the gut.

Other functions of amino acids that assist with gut health include the following:

- **Enzymes**—Made up of amino acids, enzymes are vital to our digestion and contribute to many processes throughout the body.
- **Storage and transport**—Proteins transport blood sugar, cholesterol, and other nutrients throughout the body.
- **Intestinal lining**—Amino acids strengthen the intestinal barrier, protecting against pathogens.
- **Antibody production**—Amino acids are needed to produce antibodies that the immune system uses to fight infections.
- **Collagen production**—Collagen is made from four amino acids, and it is the most abundant protein in our

bodies. It's the main structural protein in our skin, making up 70 percent of our skin's protein, but it's also in other connective tissues (muscles, bones, and tendons). It is important for gut health because it supports the intestinal wall, creating a healthy intestinal barrier.

- **Hormones and neurotransmitters**—Proteins are essential to hormone and neurotransmitter processes, which affect many bodily functions, including digestion, mood, immunity, stress response, reproductive health, and more.

The best food sources of amino acids are quality, clean animal proteins like meat, poultry, and eggs, but you can also get them through plant sources.

6. Optimize Your Diet

It's important to avoid foods that cause inflammation and contribute to a leaky gut. Start by adding in healthy whole foods. Then you can either follow an elimination diet or you can gradually remove foods with gluten, dairy, eggs, corn, and soy.

Chapter 11 includes more detail on dietary principles that can preserve and improve your health.

Elimination Diets

An elimination diet plan involves removing foods that may be causing inflammation or other symptoms, allowing the body a chance to heal. Eliminating and reintroducing foods helps you determine which foods cause symptoms or reactions. After a period of elimination (usually three to four weeks), foods are slowly reintroduced, and you monitor how your body reacts.

Elimination diets are tough. It's a huge sudden change and it's hard to determine what to eat, especially when you are on the run. Some people jump right into elimination diets. For me, it was a gradual process. I think many would agree that it is very difficult to stop eating many of your regularly eaten foods while you are in the midst of raising kids, caring for parents, racing back and forth to work, cooking, cleaning, etc. If you can do it, more power to you! I started by cutting down on gluten and dairy and adding in more vegetables and superfoods. I worked up to a completely gluten-free diet and later eliminated dairy, soy, shellfish, and eggs. I have added some dairy and eggs back in. Health coaches often recommend "adding in" at first so you become accustomed to preparing and planning healthy options. It's a gentler approach. Do what works for you.

Foods to Eliminate

Experts recommend cutting all seven top allergens at once and then adding them back in one at a time, so it becomes easy to identify what foods you react to. These allergens are:

- Gluten (wheat, barley, and rye)
- Dairy
- Soy
- Eggs
- Sugar
- Tree nuts and peanuts
- Shellfish

Nightshade vegetables are also commonly eliminated. Finned fish and sesame seeds were recently added as common allergens.

Conditions Helped by Elimination Diets

Numerous studies have demonstrated the benefit of using a food elimination diet in treating health conditions. Conditions that benefit from an elimination diet include autoimmune conditions, leaky gut syndrome, gastrointestinal symptoms, food allergies and food intolerances, attention deficit hyperactivity disorder (ADHD), migraine headaches, and skin irritations.[107]

Elimination Diet Tips

- Don't just focus on what you can't have. Do some planning and focus on what you WILL eat.
- Don't expect to feel better immediately. If you start detoxing some of the unhealthy foods, you may feel a little worse at first. Drink plenty of water and herbal teas.
- Fuel your body with nutritious foods, including fruits, vegetables, and healthy sources of protein.
- Don't skip the reintroduction phase. You may be feeling great, but the purpose of the elimination diet is to clean the slate and then test for tolerance by introducing ONE food at a time to determine what your body is reacting to.
- Once you've worked through the reintroduction period, make sure you rotate your food choices to prevent new food sensitivities from developing. Eating the same foods all the time can cause you to develop sensitivities to those foods.
- Food allergies may not be forever! Do not think you are doomed to limited food options. With time, as your gut heals and inflammation subsides, many people are able digest and tolerate more foods.
- A food journal is helpful to record what you have eaten over a given time period. In addition to food and drink intake, you should record your symptoms, how you feel emotionally, if you feel stressed, if you feel inflamed, etc. It can also be helpful to note your blood sugar and blood pressure. It's an effort initially, but it's a temporary task that can save time in the long run once you figure out what your triggers are. Some food allergies are not immediately noticeable as inflammation takes time to go down. In Chapter 11, you will learn more about food allergies and dietary considerations.

SIBO

Studies have shown that approximately 54 percent of people with hypothyroidism have small intestinal bacteria overgrowth (SIBO). Functional medicine doctors have been treating more and more people with SIBO. There is no single best treatment. You should work with a functional medicine doctor to develop an individualized treatment plan specific to your needs.

Parasite Cleanse

It's ironic that our animals are tested for parasites, and that other countries routinely test for parasites, but in the United States, our health insurance does not cover a parasite test. I personally never visited a physician that ordered a parasite test. In my opinion, the lack of parasite testing in the U.S. is irresponsible and dangerous. Parasites are at the root of a lot of different illnesses and if left untreated can lead to serious problems.

I asked for a parasite test after I learned from Dr. Izabella Wentz about the blastocystis hominis parasite and its connection with Hashimoto's disease. The blastocystis hominis parasite can make Hashimoto's worse or contribute to causing it. Many doctors consider it to be harmless. It's common in developing countries. In fact, 50 percent of people in developing countries have it. You can catch it from drinking tainted water anywhere and it is common in Mexico, which could be where I caught it. It can also be picked up by handling food or not washing hands after a bowel movement. It can happen right here in the U. S. in your own kitchen or in a restaurant.

Many of us have read horror stories about people that do parasite cleanses and huge amounts of worms come out of their bodies. I was aware that could happen, but I did a cleanse anyway. Thankfully, nothing horrifying emerged!

Blastocystis Hominis

The blastocystis hominis parasite is microscopic. It is not a long scary worm, or even a tiny worm in your body. It clings to the walls of the intestines tightly which makes it difficult to eradicate. I treated myself by going on the following supplements for three months.

- Wormwood, walnut, and clove formula (liquid tincture)
- Mimosa pudica seed (capsules)

You must be very consistent with taking the supplements and take them long enough to make the parasite let go, release from the wall, and be eliminated. It can be done in a matter of weeks or a matter of months in more resistant cases. I later asked Dr. Menashe, my primary physician to retest so that I could make sure it was gone. He said it was hard to eradicate blastocystis hominis and that he could prescribe metronidazole (Flagyl), but the test results came in and I was clean! Dr. Menashe asked how I did it and he made a note of what I had taken. He was not familiar with mimosa pudica seed. He's an excellent doctor and he's very knowledgeable, but doctors do not know everything. NO one knows everything. I just happened to have attended a parasite summit and I learned a lot about parasites, including the parasite killing herb, mimosa pudica seed. Of course, I cannot guarantee this combination would kill all parasites in everyone. This combination was effective for me, and I had no side effects. Regardless, there are many good parasite formulas available. Look for formulas that include the herbs described below.

Natural Parasite Treatments

The following items have been shown to kill parasites:

- **Clove**—Clove essential oil or the dried herb kills parasites by destroying the eggs that worms lay in the intestinal tract. It has a compound, eugenol, that is believed to dissolve the hard casing around the parasite eggs. Clove is even more powerful when combined with black walnut and wormwood.

- **Black walnut**—Black walnut hull is an effective treatment for worms and other parasites living within the human digestive system. It is an effective antiparasitic, antibacterial, and anti-fungal intestinal cleanser. It helps to push trapped parasites into your colon so they can be expelled from your body.
- **Mimosa pudica seed**—This plant is considered by many to be the best herbal treatment for parasites because it **kills the eggs** as well the adults. The seeds have a gooey fat-soluble material that sticks to everything and helps to support the entire intestinal tract. This little seed can trap parasites that have been in your gut for decades.
- **Sweet wormwood**—Also known as artemisia, sweet wormwood is an extremely bitter herb that kills parasites, including one of the most dangerous malaria parasites. It also reduces inflammation in the gut.
- **Garlic**—Garlic has powerful antimicrobial properties against parasites, bacteria, viruses, and fungi. If crushed and eaten, it can keep the parasites away and everyone else too! It also comes in capsules as the compound "allicin" which is also effective.
- **Diatomaceous earth**—Food-grade diatomaceous earth can destroy intestinal parasites, balance intestinal flora, and absorb harmful toxins.
- **Oregano oil**—Oregano oil is one of the best herbs for killing parasites and other microbes including bacteria, viruses, fungi, and even MRSA.

Treating parasites is essential to good health. Untreated parasitic infections can cause serious health problems with the digestive system and various organs. The herbs described above are helpful to the gut, instead of being harmful.

Ivermectin Medication

Ivermectin is a medication that has been safely used to treat various parasites in both humans and animals for decades. It is most well-known for treating river blindness in humans, which is caused by a parasite that gets passed to humans from black flies, mostly in Sub-Saharan Africa, but also in Central and South America. Ivermectin is a broad-spectrum anti-microbial drug with antiparasitic, antibacterial, antiviral, anti-inflammatory, and anti-cancer properties and it is well tolerated.[108] Ivermectin has dozens of other applications and is currently showing promise in studies as a treatment for cancer.[109] Other parasite medications such as Mebendazole have similar benefits but some of them can be harsh on the digestive tract. Consult your physician.

How to Avoid a "Herxheimer" Reaction

Detoxing too quickly can trigger a detox crisis, which is commonly referred to as a "Herxheimer" reaction, also known as a "herx" or "die-off" reaction. This happens when your system gets overwhelmed because pathogens that have died leave behind cellular waste and byproducts. These can come from viruses, fungus, parasites, or bacteria. This toxic waste can circulate through your bloodstream and get redistributed to organs in your body, such as the liver or brain.

This is why I recommend you start slowly and gradually increase your dose, while staying hydrated, eating clean, and giving yourself time to rest. Refer to Chapter 8 for more tips on how to manage your detox.

Schedule Stress Relief

Most of us have stressful lives. Should you just keep pushing? Not necessarily. Many of us do that to our own detriment. Let your mind and body recover. Learn to say no and ask for help.

When your body is under stress, your adrenal glands produce cortisol and other hormones to help manage the stress. The adrenal glands are very small, and they work very hard to produce enough cortisol to manage chronic stress.

Your body makes stress management a higher priority than digestion, immune modulation, and thyroid hormone production. This is not good. Normally, when stress passes quickly, your body recovers as it's designed to do. However, many of us are chronically stressed. This prolonged stress on the body results in the adrenal glands getting burned out which can cause the following negative effects:

- Slowed production of thyroid hormones
- Reduced conversion of thyroid hormone from T4 to T3 (the active form)
- Worsened leaky gut
- Increased inflammation

We all have stress in our lives, especially working single mothers. Some people take on too much. Some people have no choice. Of course, we cannot eliminate stress from our lives completely. The key is to discover which stress-relievers work for you. I personally enjoy chatting with my kids and friends, walking my dog, singing, Zumba dancing, and watching funny shows and movies. Sometimes, I take deep cleansing breaths, watch inspiring or educational videos, or meditate. When the stress at work is severe, I get away from my desk and go for a walk, prepare a meal or snack, water the garden, or spend time with my son. Skipping meals or eating the wrong food is something I have done, and it caught up with me eventually. I suggest that you include stress-relieving activities daily to prevent yourself from living in a state of chronic stress. Make the time to do it. Make the time to get outdoors, stretch, breathe, prepare healthy juices, nutritional drinks, smoothies, and salads. It only takes a few minutes. You are worth it.

Healing your gut is probably the most important part of healing autoimmune disease and many other illnesses. It is the foundation of health because your gut determines the amount of nutrients that your body absorbs. It is also the main control center for your immune system and for your neurotransmitter production. When your gut is out of balance, it can cause many problems, including inflammation, pain, allergies, mood swings, elimination problems and toxicity. On the positive side, when you have good gut health, you have better overall health, a better mood, and more energy.

CHAPTER 11

Diet, Exercise, and Metabolism

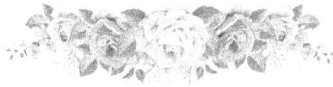

"Fat people who want to reduce should take their exercise on an empty stomach and sit down to their food out of breath … Thin people who want to get fat should do exactly the opposite and never take exercise on an empty stomach."
– Hippocrates

Food gives us pleasure and nourishment. It can give us energy or make us tired. What you eat matters! It's important to discover which way of eating works best for you. Many people with Hashimoto's follow the Autoimmune Protocol (AIP) or Paleo diet, both of which are naturally gluten-free and grain-free. I think people should do what works with them, as long as they feel well and have good thyroid lab results. Not everyone's body is the same. You should experiment and do what works for you. You should also be aware of the long-term effects. For example, following a diet that works in the short term may not be sustainable for long-term results.

Carbohydrates, fats, and proteins are macronutrients and are the three basic components of our diet. Vitamins and minerals are micronutrients that are vital to our health. Eating a healthy diet, improving your digestion, and filling your nutrient deficiencies is key to managing and overcoming this disease.

Gluten

First, we must face the truth about gluten. If you consume gluten, your antibodies may increase. There is scientific evidence showing that **a gluten-free diet results in reduced thyroid antibodies and a slightly increased vitamin D level.**[110]

I have talked with many people that do not recognize the connection between their diet and their symptoms. They continue to eat the offending foods and tell me about their symptoms, and they still don't acknowledge the connection. There are certain staples that we grew up eating such as bread, crackers, and milk. Many people just can't accept that those foods could be causing a problem. It is hard to accept for many people and I totally understand. My mother used to take me to "Dandy Donuts" in the morning when the donuts were freshly made, and the glaze was still dripping. We all have fond memories associated with food.

It took me several years to acknowledge that gluten was a serious problem for me. It was not clear in the beginning (before I was diagnosed). We all get bloated or sleepy after eating sometimes. I noticed I would crash after lunch at work if I ate carbs or gluten with my lunch. I started by cutting back. I had a few experiences dining out where I felt horrible afterward. One was at a Japanese Hibachi restaurant. Soy sauce can be made gluten-free but regular soy sauce has wheat. I had severe abdominal pain and bloating afterwards. I was incapacitated for the rest of the night. I had to quit eating Japanese and Chinese food due to most dishes having both wheat and soy.

It finally became clear to me that I was gluten intolerant, not just sensitive. Over time, the reactions worsened. After eating it, I would be sleepy, bloated, and sometimes constipated. Sometimes, I would have body aches and experience blurry vision. Later it got worse, and I experienced sharp abdominal pain and malaise and then I would fall asleep. When I eliminated gluten from my diet, I noticed a huge improvement. My bloating went down, my energy increased, and I felt more mental clarity.

Several years into this discovery process, one of my favorite doctors, Dr. Cesar Holgado, ran a very comprehensive gut panel. I really appreciated that he was able to run this panel. The results showed that I was allergic to 31 different gliadins. Gliadins are proteins that exist in wheat. He said that I was so allergic, that I shouldn't even walk into a bakery! That hit home.

I was extra careful after that round of blood work. That test confirmed without a doubt that my body was extremely sensitive to gluten. I strictly avoided gluten and became that pain in the neck person when ordering in restaurants. I even ordered new lipsticks that were gluten free.

Why Gluten is Harmful

When gluten is eaten by someone with leaky gut, gluten molecules seep through the intestinal walls and the immune system mistakes the gluten for thyroid cells and then targets thyroid cells. This may sound strange to some people, especially if you are not familiar with leaky gut syndrome and autoimmune disease. However, I think most people suffering with chronic illness have heard about leaky gut and the importance of healing the gut.

Dr. Tom O'Bryan is a world expert on gluten and how it impacts people's health. He is an internationally recognized speaker that specializes in non-celiac gluten sensitivity, celiac disease, and the development of autoimmune diseases. I have attended multiple events where he was either the host or a guest speaker. In 2013, he hosted the Gluten Summit and interviewed experts on gluten from all the over the world. I listened to 26 of the foremost experts present the science on gluten. I must admit it was depressing. The science demonstrated that the immune system attacks the thyroid when you consume gluten, especially in people with leaky gut. Your immune system remembers pathogens you have been exposed to (such as viruses, bacteria, etc.) and thus defends you. The problem is that the immune system sometimes mistakes other substances, such as gluten or dairy proteins, for cells in your bodily tissues. In the case of Hashimoto's, the thyroid is attacked. With other autoimmune diseases, other tissues are attacked. This is called molecular mimicry.

An easy (and free) way to test for gluten sensitivity is to stop eating it completely—and I mean 100 percent for at least 30 days, but preferably three months, and then reintroduce it. Note how you feel while you are off it, and how you feel when you eat it again. Do you feel tired, moody, bloated, cramped, headaches, body aches, general inflammation, or changes in bowel habits? Doing this should determine if you have gluten sensitivity and if so, you should stop eating it because it may be causing more damage than you are aware of.

If you are unsure or want to verify by lab work, ask your doctor to order blood tests. There are specific tests for non-celiac gluten sensitivity. There is a test for celiac disease and some doctors stop there, but you don't want it to progress to celiac disease. You should be tested for "anti-gliadin antibodies." Request the IgG anti-gliadin antibodies test.

Eat Clean

Eat clean whole foods. Avoid foods with pesticides, herbicides, and fungicides. Avoid additives, preservatives, artificial sweeteners, and colors. The shorter the ingredient list, the better. Keep in mind that the ingredients are listed in order of what the product has the most of.

Eat organic fruits and vegetables as much as possible. You can also shop at your local farms and ask them about what they use on their crops. I have found several farms in my area that do not use pesticides. If you cannot purchase all organic, use the Environmental Working Group's "Dirty Dozen" and "Clean Fifteen" lists as a guide. The "Dirty Dozen" lists the fruits and vegetables with the highest level of pesticide residue. The list includes spinach, celery, strawberries, peaches, cherries, grapes, blueberries, tomatoes, pears, apples, potatoes, and sweet bell peppers. These are the fruits and vegetables that are most important to buy organic.

The "Clean Fifteen" list the fruits and vegetables with the lowest levels of pesticide residue. You can download both lists and other materials, including a guide to additives, on the EWG website. The EWG is a wonderful organization that fights against the use of pesticides on baby food and much more.[111]

Food Allergies

The foods we eat can have an enormous impact on our health. Be aware of your food allergies or sensitivities. There are two types of food allergies. One is immediate and obvious. You may experience itchy throat and mouth, maybe even constriction of the esophagus. You may break out in hives or a rash. You may have nausea, cramps, feel bloated, experience indigestion, gas, and acid reflux. These allergies can be identified by an IgE test.

The other type of allergy is trickier. It could be the next day or several days later that your body shows signs of a reaction, and the connection may be unclear. You might experience overall inflammation or digestive issues such as constipation, diarrhea, cramping. You may have a post-nasal drip, congestion, coughing, acne, eczema, joint pain, headache, brain fog, anxiety, depression, fatigue, and insomnia. Some tests measure IgG antibodies but these are not considered accurate. Skin prick tests or an elimination diet are known to be more accurate.

Eating foods that trigger allergies or sensitivities can also trigger your autoimmune condition and result in increased thyroid antibodies which leads to the destruction of your thyroid tissue. Most people experience a significant reduction in digestive symptoms, brain fog, skin breakouts, and pain, simply by eliminating the foods they are sensitive to. Some people also have a significant reduction in thyroid antibodies.

Although food allergies can be very limiting, with some effort, many of them can be improved. I have resolved some of my food allergies and I know of other people that have resolved theirs as well. There are several things you can try:

- Eliminate the offending food(s) for at least three months
- Heal your gut—See Chapter 10 for guidance
- Take custom allergy drops—Sublingual desensitization therapy treats food and environmental allergies and intolerances

I visited a naturopathic wellness center that specializes in *sublingual desensitization*. They have practiced this method for over 30 years, and it has proven to be safe and effective. There are no injections required. This treatment is safer and more convenient than injection therapy. The process involves getting a series of skin prick tests on your upper arm, after which custom homeopathic desensitization allergy drops are created for you. I went through this process and took the custom drops for several months and then kind of forgot about it as I was very busy. Later, I started to notice that my allergies were virtually gone, including pollen and dogs!

Goitrogens

You may have heard that you should avoid goitrogenic foods if you have a thyroid condition, but this is only partially true. Not all goitrogenic foods are the same. Cruciferous vegetables generally do not pose a problem for people with Hashimoto's, especially if they are cooked. Cooking or lightly steaming (or fermenting) them deactivates and breaks down the iodine-blocking component.

The two goitrogens to completely avoid are **soy** and **canola**. Most soy and canola crops are genetically modified. Soy is both goitrogenic and estrogenic. It blocks the activity of the TPO enzyme and has been linked to the development of autoimmune thyroiditis. It interferes with the absorption of thyroid hormones. Soy is a xenoestrogen and can affect your estrogen levels. Estrogen dominance can trigger Hashimoto's and PCOS. If you have Hashimoto's, you should avoid all soy foods, and soy ingredients in supplements and personal care products.[112] Soy is hidden is many products.

Blood Sugar

No matter what age you are or what stage of Hashimoto's you are in, blood sugar balance is very important. Many of us, including me, take it for granted when we are young. However, as you age and eventually approach menopause, blood sugar becomes a problem for many of us.

Did you know that diabetes affects up to **30 percent** of people with Hashimoto's?[113]

On the *Open Your Eyes* podcast (number one podcast in Optometry) with Dr. Kerry Gelb, it was revealed by internist Dr.

Ted Naiman that **52% of Americans are diabetic or pre-diabetic** and that **100% of diabetics have a fatty liver.** A buildup of fat in your liver can increase your sugar levels. Dr. Naiman, author of *The P:E Diet*, explained that the best way to reverse fatty liver is to simply lose fat. He says it's possible to lose the fat in the liver within weeks on a strict diet.

When you ingest sugar, the pancreas releases insulin to lower the levels of glucose in the blood. These surges in insulin can cause blood sugar levels to drop too low, which subsequently causes cravings for more carbohydrate-rich foods. This can become a vicious cycle, causing your blood sugar levels to surge up and crash down, creating a strain on your body. Stabilizing your blood sugar can help in the effort to reverse Hashimoto's.[114]

Exercise is one of the best ways to lower your blood sugar. Working out helps to improve your circulation and support your insulin and blood sugar balance. If diet and lifestyle changes do not help you to balance your insulin and glucose levels, you should work with your physicians to find a working combination of medications and/or supplements.

Two supplements strongly supported by research are **berberine** and **Myo-inositol**. If you are pre-diabetic or suffering with diabetes type 2, you may want to consider using these supplements to restore normal thyroid function, balance blood sugar, and help address insulin resistance.[115] See Chapter 13 for more information about these nutraceuticals and Chapter 16 for an advanced holistic treatment that lowers blood sugar substantially.

Satiety

Dr. Gelb asked Dr. Naiman to identify the top reason for people not losing weight. The number one reason is not doing enough exercise. The number two reason is not eating enough macronutrients to make you feel satisfied or satiated. Dr. Naiman suggests tracking your exercise and your macronutrient intake (i.e., carbs, protein, and fat).

Proteins create the highest satiety per calorie. Satiety is also achieved by eating foods with fiber and micronutrients like potassium, calcium, folate, and vitamin C. However, when you eat foods with refined sugar, carbohydrates, alcohol, and unhealthy oils, you are consuming empty calories without satiety. This can lead to overeating because you do not have full satiety.

Metabolism

Many people with hypothyroidism and Hashimoto's struggle with a slow metabolism. Hashimoto's is the leading cause of hypothyroidism, which is a metabolic disorder because it results in lower production of hormones that are important for your metabolism. Even mild hypothyroidism is linked to an increased risk of obesity, weight gain, and insulin resistance.

Your metabolic rate is determined by your age, weight, and activity level. Genes also factor into the equation. Metabolism in adults declines at a rate of about 10 percent each decade. Insulin resistance can slow your metabolism even more, worsening your chances of losing weight. When menopause begins, it becomes even harder.

Things that boost metabolism include:

- Movement—Regular exercise helps you to burn calories and increase lean muscle mass. All exercise boosts metabolism but strength training and high-intensity interval training gives an extra boost to your metabolism.
- Eat regular meals—Starvation diets make the body slow down the rate at which it uses energy.
- Rest—While you sleep, your body is busy repairing tissue and removing waste products which contributes to overall health and your metabolism.

- Improve liver health—Your liver function is key to the conversion of glucose and thyroid hormones. Having a fatty liver slows your metabolism.
- Detox periodically and avoid toxins.
- Limit sweets and processed foods.
- Eat enough protein to help your body maintain muscle mass.
- Stay hydrated.

See Chapter 13 to learn about nutraceuticals that help with metabolism and insulin resistance.

Exercise

Exercise is one of the best preventative medicines. It energizes you and boosts your mood by increasing your endorphins. It's great for your heart and it stimulates your circulation, helping your lymphatic system to eliminate toxins. It's so important to work your muscles, especially your core muscles. Our muscles and bones weaken as we age. You must strengthen and tone your muscles and do weight-bearing exercise to maintain bone density.

Work your core and twist. It helps your liver to move it by twisting the abdominals! Lengthen and strengthen your spine. They say you are as young as your spine. No one likes an aching back and having trouble bending over to pick things up or doing household chores. Remember, strong body, strong mind. Challenge yourself and be consistent. You will love the feeling of being stronger, more flexible, and more energetic.

Many people with autoimmune disease experience more soreness than the average person after working out. I must admit being discouraged by this, especially after shoulder surgery and a terrible fall that damaged both of my knees. I was very inflamed, and I suffered with stiffness and pain for a long time.

Squats, lunges, jumping, and running were out of the question. However, I've had some treatments and I do modified workouts that help me maintain my strength and flexibility.

There are many types of workouts you can do that do not cause you pain. You may not be able to keep up with classes at the gym and weightlifting can make you very sore if you are not very careful. However, you can gradually work your way up to some of those gym workouts or you can choose to perform a variety of other exercises that work for you. If walking is your cardio of choice, your step count should be at least 8,000 steps per day, and it's even better to get 10,000–12,000 steps.

If you don't feel like exercising, just do five minutes. You can commit to five minutes. After you get moving, you will probably want to keep going. I personally do not like going to the gym too often because of time limitations and germ concerns. I do a variety of exercise routines at home. I enjoy stretching, dance, and aerobics videos. I do a series of dumbbell and bar workouts for upper body. I go on power walks. I use stretchy bands, weighted balls, and I even have a swivel thing I stand on and just twist side to side.

My favorite workouts videos are from Zumba Sulu and Denise Austin. Denise is a career professional and her workouts are varied and effective. She has many short videos so you can do five, 10, 20, or 30 minutes. You really feel it, but you don't get sore! I also love Zumba Sulu. He has great music and fun, low impact dance moves that give you a great workout.

My naturopathic doctor, Dr. Glenn Gero, gave me a goal of 300 minutes of exercise per week. That is about 45 minutes per day. He suggested logging the minutes in a calendar. He also advised me that high intensity internal training (HIIT) has been shown to improve thyroid hormone levels.[116]

Diets

"The usual justification for eating extra meals is that it keeps the metabolism 'revved up' so that weight loss is easier. There is, however, very little hard evidence that supports this idea, and a fair amount that disputes it."
– Dr. Andrew Weil

Several diets have been reported to improve Hashimoto's and other autoimmune conditions. They include:

Whole food, plant-based (WFPB) diet—A WFPB diet has been shown to improve symptoms of autoimmune disease and also helps to prevent the development of autoimmune conditions. This diet helps by decreasing inflammation and by supporting the health of your gut microbiome.

A WFPB diet provides a high level of nutrients and antioxidants, has no adverse side effects, and is associated with other health benefits such as cardiometabolic health, healthy weight, and longevity.[243, 244] Additional benefits are associated with a gluten-free plant-based diet.[245]

Mediterranean diet (MD)—The Mediterranean diet consists of small amounts of red meat, low to moderate amounts of poultry and fish, and plenty of fruit, vegetables, whole grains, and legumes with olive oil, which serves as an important source of monounsaturated fatty acids (MUFA). The plant polyphenols have been shown to reduce insulin resistance and lower cardiovascular risk.[117] The MD diet has been shown to be beneficial for people with endocrine disorders, including thyroid disease.[118]

Paleo diet—A simple diet based on how people ate in the past before processed food existed. This diet consists of local, organic, non-GMO products like fruits, vegetables, nuts, and seeds, plus fish and grass-fed beef. This diet is high in protein and fiber, contains an average amount of fat, and is low in carbs.[119] The paleo diet has been shown to reduce thyroid antibodies and improve thyroid hormone levels.[120]

Autoimmune Paleo (AIP) diet—The AIP diet involves identifying and removing the foods that cause inflammation in your gut. This diet is very restrictive and requires you to eliminate several foods. You have the option to eliminate foods one at a time as your body adjusts. You can choose to eliminate one category of foods per week (for example, dairy, grains, nightshade vegetables, or processed foods). After you follow the AIP diet strictly for 30 to 90 days, you can reintroduce foods one at a time to see if your body reacts. For example, when reintroducing dairy, you might start with a serving of low-fat yogurt or milk. Consume a serving every day for three days. If you do not notice a negative reaction, you add other richer dairy products in phases and write down any observations.[121]

Specific carbohydrate diet (SCD)—The specific carbohydrate diet has been shown to be very helpful to people with digestive conditions such as inflammatory bowel disease, Crohn's disease, ulcerative colitis, celiac disease, diverticulitis, cystic fibrosis, and chronic diarrhea. It has also been shown to be helpful for those with autism. It is a grain-free diet that allows some carbs and bans others, based on how hard they are to digest. The intention is to reduce leftover undigested carbohydrates that cause overgrowth of bad bacteria.[122]

Diets free of gluten, soy, dairy, and/or iodine—where these foods are eliminated.

Note: Carbs should not be completely avoided. Essential body parts, including the brain, muscles (during exercise), and various organs, require carbohydrates for optimal functioning.

Dietary Guidelines

Regardless of the diet you choose to follow, here are some general principles:

- Aim for nutrient density. Eat plenty of organic fruit and vegetables, green drinks, pasture-raised or organic protein sources, mineral rich bone broth, fermented foods, and gelatins. These are all foods that are chock full of healing and beneficial nutrients.
- Make fresh green smoothies with protein powder, fresh or frozen fruit, and "superfood" or green powder for five to seven meals per week.
- Eat a variety of foods and rotate them often. If you have leaky gut, eating the same food all the time, no matter how healthy it is, can lead to you becoming sensitive to that food.
- If you are still using regular table salt, change your salt to sea salt or Himalayan pink salt, which both contain 80 trace minerals.
- Eliminate industrially processed food (i.e., processed grains, cereals, bagels, pasta, crackers, cookies, chips, etc.).
- Eliminate or reduce the most common reactive foods like gluten, dairy, soy, eggs, caffeine, and sugar.
- Strive to eat 75 percent vegetables and 25 percent healthy protein (lean meat, fish, or fowl) per meal.
- Eat low glycemic foods to try to maintain blood sugar balance. Blood sugar imbalances are often a problem with those with Hashimoto's. Eating a low-GI diet can help to maintain steady energy, prevent mood swings, and reduce the autoimmune attack on the thyroid.
- Include a small amount of healthy fat from sources such as coconut, avocado, and seeds (such as chia, flax, and hemp) to support hair, skin, balanced blood sugar, brain health, and cardiovascular health.

- Include omega-3 fatty acids either from wild-caught fish or from vegan omega-3 supplements.
- Include pastured, grass-fed butter if you can tolerate dairy. It's a nutritional powerhouse of vitamins A, D, K2, and heart-disease preventing CLA (conjugated linoleic acid). The vitamin K2 in pastured butter helps with bone and tooth maintenance.
- Avoid pesticides as much as possible. They damage the gut and your health in general. Glyphosate for example, has been shown to increase the risk of cancer and other diseases.
- Hydrate with clean, filtered water or spring water. Some people choose to buy alkaline water, structured water, or hydrogen water. Hydrogen water has especially impressive therapeutic benefits.

Home Cooking

If you don't cook, I suggest you try to prepare your own meals. It's much cheaper and you can control what you are consuming. Restaurant meals typically contain a lot of hidden fat and salt. You can also use clean non-toxic cookware and utensils and avoid toxins in takeout containers. Simply learning the basics of preparing clean protein sources and sautéing or steaming vegetables can help you make plenty of combinations. Cooking is not that difficult. It doesn't have to be gourmet. It's home cooking! Seasoning with salt, pepper, and garlic makes most things delicious. There are also plenty of seasoning blends with herbs and spices that taste great. If you learn, you'll be so proud of yourself and so satisfied with all the money you save.

I have always been a foodie. I enjoy cooking AND dining out. However, when you are trying to eat clean and you must avoid certain allergens and unhealthy foods, your choice of restaurants narrows. I have a certain number of places I frequent, and I like to try new places occasionally. I have a son with autism, and he prefers to eat the same foods at the same places. He and I spend lots of time together, so that limits my usual adventures in dining, but I encourage him to try new things. Occasionally, I come up with a dish that he loves, and I am able to expand his palate a bit more.

As your kids get older (if you have kids), I suggest that you encourage them to pay for their own restaurant meals so that they can learn how much money is wasted on eating out. This made my sons want to cook their own meals. It costs a fraction of the price of restaurant meals, and you can control the ingredients and cleanliness, and especially the types of fats that are used. Restaurants use a lot of butter and oil and some of these oils are likely GMO and reused repeatedly. Wouldn't you rather have a fresh dish with a carefully measured amount of grass-fed butter, avocado oil, coconut oil, or quality extra virgin olive oil?

Stick with it!

Even if you are discouraged and confused, don't give up! That's one thing I want to convey to my esteemed readers—to never give up. Please don't just start eating gluten (or other allergens) again and say to yourself, "Forget it! I don't feel good anyway, so I'm just going to eat what I want!" It's a tempting thought but it's not going to work. If you get off track for a meal, or a day or week, just get back on track. It takes time to heal. Be patient with yourself.

They are a lot of actions that will elevate how you feel over time. Stay positive and keep taking the steps outlined in this book. It's absolutely worth it. If you are fatigued, simply getting your energy back is worth the effort!

When your energy returns, your pain is gone, your mood is happy, and you're bopping around and getting things done, it's a wonderful feeling. It's also hugely rewarding if you restore your thyroid health so that it's producing healthy amounts of thyroid hormone on its own.

CHAPTER 12

Iodine Controversy Clarified

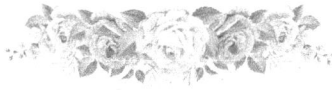

"There are in fact two things, science and opinion. The former begets knowledge, the latter ignorance."
— Hippocrates

Iodine is a trace mineral and an essential nutrient. Iodine is critical to human health. It is essential to normal growth and development.

The largest amount of iodine in your body is found in the endocrine system. Iodine is needed by the thyroid gland to produce thyroid hormones Thyroxine (T4) and Triiodothyronine (T3), which are secreted into your blood and then transported and utilized by every tissue in your body. Thyroid hormone is necessary for the cells of your organs and tissues to function properly. It helps your body use energy, stay warm, and allows your heart, brain, and other organs to work optimally.

Iodine is in many foods, added to some types of salt, and is available as a dietary supplement. Iodine is abundant in the sea and thus plentiful in seafood, kelp, and seaweed. However, iodine levels in foods that grow in soil depend on the amount of iodine that exists in the soil.

It is important to have enough iodine, but not too much if you have thyroid disease. There are conflicting opinions and misconceptions about iodine supplementation for thyroid disease. It is a complex subject. Many people have taken huge doses of iodine and although many of them felt better for some time, their thyroid antibodies skyrocketed. I have examined multiple sources on both sides of the debate, including two comprehensive reviews of the literature. In the last few years, new scientific studies have become available that clarify how iodine affects people with Hashimoto's and hypothyroidism. My goal is to provide an objective and up-to-date summary.

Essential to Know

Most People with Hashimoto's Disease are NOT Deficient in Iodine.
According to Dr. Izabella Wentz, "most people with Hashimoto's are not deficient in iodine."
Based on a review of the literature, the only people who should supplement with iodine are those that have a lab-validated iodine deficiency. [123]

Iodine is a controversial issue in relation to hypothyroidism and Hashimoto's. In this chapter, you will learn the flawed hypothesis that resulted in many thyroid patients taking very large doses of iodine supplements. You will also learn about the risks of taking excess iodine.

For the sake of your thyroid tissue, it is important to get this right. It's essential to understanding the following:

- If you have Hashimoto's disease, iodine supplementation is highly likely to increase your thyroid antibodies. This in effect causes the immune system to attack and damage the thyroid more over time.
- If you have Hashimoto's disease, you may feel much better after you begin taking an iodine supplement, but later on down the road, you will likely feel much worse. This is a temporary effect due to the iodine supplement causing the thyroid to quickly excrete extra thyroid hormone, thus raising your T3 and T4 levels. However, over time it exacerbates Hashimoto's disease. The destruction of thyroid cells accelerates, causing significant damage to the thyroid gland.
- If you are selenium-deficient, taking iodine can cause a thyroid storm. This can make the immune system overactive in your thyroid and cause an autoimmune flare-up.
- If you are iodine-deficient (based on a valid lab test), and you decide to supplement, there are a few things to consider. Caution should be exercised. Consider the iodine in what you are eating. Selenium levels MUST be healthy AND you should not start while detoxing.

Iodine supplementation has been shown to shrink goiters. This is only in cases where there is a lab-verified iodine deficiency causing the goiter*.

---

* Mandatory salt iodization programs have essentially eliminated iodine deficiency in most industrialized countries which affects 70 percent of the world's population. However, now there are problems associated with too much iodine. **Increased iodine intake is associated with increasing numbers of thyroid diseases including Hashimoto's disease, thyroid cancer, simple goiter, and toxic nodular goiter.**

Iodine Supplementation Triggers Hashimoto's Disease

Dr. Datis Kharrazian was among the very first to say NO IODINE for Hashimoto's. There are now many doctors and medical institutions warning about iodine's effect on those with Hashimoto's.

For example:

- The **Mayo Clinic** agrees with not supplementing with iodine for Hashimoto's disease, and states that it could be harmful.[124]
- The American Thyroid Association warns against using doses of more than 500 mcg per day for the general public and cautioned that doses above 1100 mcg may cause thyroid dysfunction. People with Hashimoto's are sensitive to even smaller doses.[125]
- A study published in the *Journal of Clinical Endocrinology and Metabolism* examined the relationship between iodine intake and hypothyroidism. They studied patients in Japan where dietary intake of iodine is high. They found that there is a reversible type of hypothyroidism based on biopsies of thyroid tissue. With this type of hypothyroidism, **thyroid function returned to normal by simply restricting iodine intake for three weeks**. When those people were given iodine again, the hypothyroidism returned. In contrast, the people with the *irreversible* type of hypothyroidism already had more severe destruction on their thyroid gland.[126]
- A review in the *International Journal of Molecular Sciences* states that excess iodine intake is a well-established environmental risk factor for the development of autoimmune thyroid diseases (ATD), especially for susceptible individuals. Iodine supplementation increases thyroid antibodies if you have Hashimoto's and can worsen your condition by increasing the destruction of thyroid

cells. In addition, excess iodine in thyroid cells can result in elevated levels of oxidative stress, which leads to harmful lipid oxidation and thyroid tissue injuries.[127]

People that suffer with autoimmune disease typically have a lot of oxidative stress and inflammation. Iodine promotes oxidation and inflammation. Oxidative stress can lead to many problems, including organ and tissue damage. If you have Hashimoto's disease and you eat foods with a lot of iodine or take iodine supplements, it **reduces** your body's ability to make thyroid hormone over time. You will likely need thyroid replacement. This process could take one year, or it could take 10 years.

It's tricky because many people with Hashimoto's or hypothyroidism report feeling better when they start to take iodine. Why? Because it makes the thyroid **spill thyroid hormone** faster than normal which can increase the T4 and T3 levels. This can help increase energy and metabolism. The problem is that when this process is continued over time, it reduces the thyroid's ability to produce thyroid hormone on its own. The second reason you might feel better is because your body did need some iodine and you feel better. This does not mean you should ignore potential risks and continue taking it long term. This practice speeds up the autoimmune process and progresses the disease.

The Controversy

People are very passionate about this subject. Many people make strong claims based on anecdotal evidence, blogs, and websites, but do not cite any peer-reviewed studies to back up their claims. I have consulted with many respected sources and clinical studies for information on the iodine debate. My goal is to be objective and share the science as well as my personal experience, which corroborated the science.

I took iodine. I felt better. My antibodies went up. I went off it. My antibodies went down. I felt just the same.

Still, I have compassion for those people that have been advised to take iodine and then continue supplementing with iodine because it helped them escape the crippling fatigue caused by hypothyroidism. However, just because something helps you feel better temporarily (e.g., opioid pain medications), it doesn't mean it is good for you long term. I want people to be aware of the long-term effects.

Thyroid Mega-Dosing Study

The science I describe below influenced women and men all over to start taking large doses of iodine supplements, up to 60 mg. Iodine mega dosing became popular in 1997 after Dr. Guy Abraham, a former professor of obstetrics and gynecology at UCLA, started the "Iodine Project." His company, Optimox Corporation, **makes** Iodoral, the tablet form of Lugol's solution (which combines iodine and potassium iodide). It sounds like a conflict of interest to me but here's what happened.

Dr. Abraham recruited two respected family practice physicians, Dr. Jorge Flechas (in 2000) in North Carolina and Dr. David Brownstein (in 2003) in Michigan to run clinical studies providing high doses of Iodoral. Their hypothesis was that the body needs 12.5 mg of iodine daily, which is **over 80 times** the Reference Daily Intake (RDI) of 150 mcg.

Iodine levels were assessed in a way that was based on a faulty hypothesis.

Dr. Abraham suggested that the whole body has sufficient iodine if a person excretes **90 percent** of the iodine they have ingested in their urine. He created an iodine-loading test where one takes 50 mg of Iodoral (iodine/potassium iodide), and then collects their urine over the next 24 hours. He claimed that the majority of people retain a large amount of the 50 mg dose. He said that many subjects required 50 mg per day for several months before they excreted 90 percent of it.

His work was widely popularized by Dr. Flechas and Dr. Brownstein, among others that jumped on the bandwagon. I remember hearing about it from many sources, but I was suspicious after the way my body had reacted. Maybe that experience was the universe protecting me. I had also researched both sides of the debate and found some warnings. There were strong opinions on both sides. Many people started taking Lugol's solution, many of them without medical supervision, desperately trying to feel better.

Inaccurate Iodine Loading Test Results

The high-dose iodine practice was challenged by Dr. Alan Gaby in an editorial in the *Townsend Letter* in 2005.[128]

Dr. Gaby described the iodine-loading test used by Dr. Abraham and colleagues and asked questions regarding the test's validity. After the patient takes 50 mg of iodine/potassium iodide, the patient is considered to be iodine-deficient if less than 90 percent of the 50 mg dose is excreted in the urine. They thought that a deficient person would retain iodine in their tissues, rather than excreting it in their urine. According to the literature of a laboratory that offers this test, a whopping **92–98 percent of patients who took the iodine loading test were found deficient in iodine**. This result is extraordinarily high which makes it suspect. It's highly unlikely that those numbers are accurate given that the average American diet is sufficient in iodine. This test was also proven wrong by a 2016 study at the University of Michigan which found that **only 11.6 percent** (2001–2004) to **13.2** percent (2009–2012) of women in the U.S. have low iodine levels.[129]

According to Dr. Gaby, the validity of the test is based on the assumption that the average person can absorb 90 percent of a

50 mg dose AND that the iodine excreted is considered accurately measured when testing only the urine and not the feces.

The **first flaw** is presuming a human can absorb 90 percent of a mega-dose of iodine.

The **second flaw** is presuming that people are failing to excrete 90 percent of the iodine in the urine not because their tissues are soaking it up, but because a lot of the iodine is **coming out in the feces**. There is no reason to assume that a 50 mg dose of iodine, which is at least 250 times the typical daily intake, can be almost completely absorbed by the average person. In fact, in a study with cows that were fed greater than normally ingested amounts of iodine (72 to 161 mg per day), the cows excreted approximately **50 percent** of the administered dose in the feces.

Dr. Gaby also pointed out that Dr. Lugol used high doses of the iodine and potassium iodide compound primarily to treat infections, but not as routine nutritional support for the average person. He also cited a review article stating that doctors in the 1920s and 1930s widely used potassium iodine, and many patients died of side effects, especially pulmonary edema, and associated heart failure.

According to the Weston Price review of the debate, the Abraham protocol is associated with a risk of adverse reactions and should only be done under the supervision of a physician experienced with the protocol. If taking iodine in milligram doses, the treatment protocol should include a comprehensive nutritional program that includes appropriate amounts of selenium, magnesium, and omega-3 fatty acids, and the patient should be closely monitored for detox reactions.

Iodine Testing

There are four types of tests for iodine levels. They all have problems with accuracy.

- Urine test: This is the test performed by most doctors to determine the iodine level
- Blood test: This is known to be accurate for testing iodine levels, but most labs don't do this type of testing
- Patch test: This is not known for being very accurate. It involves drawing a 2 x 2 patch on your forearm using a 2 percent tincture of iodine. If you are not iodine deficient, the patch should not fade until 24 hours have passed. If you are deficient in iodine, the patch should disappear in less time. If you have a severe iodine deficiency, the patch begins to fade or disappears in 12 hours or less.
- Urine-loading test: You take 50 mg of iodine and then collect all your urine over the next 24 hours before sending a sample of urine to the lab. The 50 mg dose of iodine is a very high dose. It is not considered to cause any permanent health issues, but I had a severe reaction after taking a 12.5 mg ioderal pill. If you are concerned about any negative effects, talk to your practitioner to see if it's the right iodine test for you. If you have hyperthyroidism or Graves' disease, this test is contraindicated and should **not** be performed.

Iodine Overdose Reactions

Dr. Izabella Wentz said, "As a pharmacist, I am often reminded that the only difference between a medicine and a poison is the dose." She says that physiological doses of iodine (that is, an amount close to what is **normally produced** in the body) can improve thyroid function. However, research shows that excessive supplemental doses of iodine can trigger **and** worsen Hashimoto's in people who are genetically predisposed to Hashimoto's and may have certain weaknesses, such as a selenium deficiency.[130]

Side effects of excessive iodine intake include severe acne, headaches, allergic reactions, metallic taste in the mouth, and parotid gland swelling.

My Reaction to Iodoral

I was in the middle of six months of EDTA chelation when Dr. Jerk gave me a 12.5 mg pill of Iodoral for the purpose of testing my iodine level. I took it and had a severe reaction. I was very emotional and distressed. I was in pain, had crushing headaches, and I was breaking out in horrible acne, like I never had experienced in the past. While I acknowledge that my reaction could potentially have been worse because I was undergoing chelation treatment, there is no way I would ever take a high dose of iodine again. It was fortunate however in the respect that I had a healthy fear of iodine supplementation and that I didn't get swept up in the megadose fervor.

It was about 10 years later after hearing such positive feedback on Global Healing's "Detoxadine" that I finally decided to try an iodine supplement. I found evidence that iodine consumption helps to detox the other harmful halogens, such as fluoride, chloride, and bromide, and even toxic metals like lead, aluminum, and mercury. This time, it was a much lower dose and a product made by a company I trusted. I began taking one drop of Detoxadine nascent iodine daily in 2019 and gradually increased up to three drops a day which provides 1950 mcg of iodine, which equals 1.95 mg. I quickly noticed an increase in my energy level. I also started to have more mental clarity. Over time, it also seemed to boost my immunity because I did not catch Covid-19 even though I was in direct contact with Covid-infected people several times.

However, after getting my blood work done two years later, my TPO antibody result was higher than had ever been measured before, at 213. While many people have antibody tests in the thousands, my highest number had been 144 when I was first diagnosed, but I had gotten it down to low numbers such as 27, 40, and 60. It was always under 100 since I was first diagnosed and started treating myself. I stopped taking the iodine and retested. My TPO antibodies went down to 35! Normal would be 0–35 so I just made it into in normal range. Would I ever take iodine again? I don't know. If I had a low level, I would use it only temporarily and cautiously, and monitor my antibodies.

Recommendations

Typically, it is easy to get enough iodine in our diet. It exists in many foods, including seaweed, cod, tuna, eggs, cheese, yogurt, turkey breast, iodized salt, spinach, lentils, quinoa, potatoes, and beans. It is advised to avoid kelp and seaweed products because the amount of iodine they contain are not always clearly measurable.

If you are currently taking an iodine supplement, check your antibodies. If they are elevated, I suggest stopping the iodine and retesting a few months later. Consult a healthcare provider that is aware of the risks of taking iodine with Hashimoto's if possible.

If you're not taking iodine and you test low in it, and your doctor suggests that you take a supplement, I recommend Detoxadine by Global Healing. It is certified organic nascent iodine created from salt deposits located more than 7,000 feet below the earth's surface, shielded from pollutants. It is a liquid which makes it easier to control your dosage. You can start with one drop and go up to three drops maximum. After a few months, have your thyroid antibodies checked. If they have increased, I would suggest stopping the iodine. That is what I did. After I stopped taking the iodine, I didn't experience any negative effects.

Although my energy increased after I started using Detoxadine, it did not go down when I stopped the iodine. Perhaps I was iodine deficient when I started and maybe I corrected that deficiency. I discovered later that soil in New Jersey is low in both iodine and selenium, so it is conceivable that I had a deficiency. I suggest that you do a search to find out if the area you live in has low levels of iodine or selenium in the soil.

As I mentioned previously, the accuracy of iodine tests is not optimal, but you can work with your physician to determine if you have a real deficiency. Perhaps a temporary course of iodine in low doses would help to detox the halogens from your thyroid and boost your energy. Just remember: Long-term iodine supplementation leads to increased thyroid antibodies and destruction of the thyroid gland's tissue.

If you supplement with iodine, I recommend that you get lab work to check your thyroid antibodies so that you know how it is affecting you. Just the same as you would do if you took a certain medication, especially medications that carry risks and require monitoring.

Lastly, consider this quote from Sayer Ji's conclusion regarding iodine supplementation for Hashimoto's:

> "If your functional medicine practitioner, nutritionist, naturopathic doctor, or alternative medicine provider recommends that you supplement with supra-physiological doses of iodine—or that you incorporate massive sea vegetables into your diet to boost thyroid function—ask them for the peer-reviewed study supporting this practice. My bet is that they will come up empty.
>
> So, why are people so invested in iodine? According to the Thyroid Pharmacist, Dr. Isabella Wentz, people may experience a short-term *artificial* increase in energy after beginning an iodine supplement. Dr. Wentz fleshes out a probable mechanism, whereby their newfound energy is derived from iodine-induced thyroid tissue destruction and the liberation of thyroid hormone into the circulation."[131]

CHAPTER 13

Healing Nutraceuticals

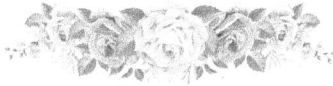

"I believe the best way to activate genius within the
immune system is by ingesting certain superherbs
and superfoods, taking probiotics and cultured
foods, minimizing toxic food exposure by eating pure
organic raw-living foods, and making appropriate
healthy lifestyle improvements."
— David Wolfe

Nutraceuticals are products derived from food sources that
provide both nutritional and medicinal benefits. These products
include dietary supplements, herbal products, and vitamins. They
contain a high concentration of bioactive compounds, derived
from natural sources, and assist in the prevention and treatment
of disease.

Nutraceuticals can improve health, delay the aging process, prevent chronic diseases, increase life expectancy, and support the structure and functioning of the body. They are also used in the prevention and treatment of mental health issues and disorders.

The term "nutraceutical" was coined in 1989 by Stephen DeFelice who is the founder and chairperson of the Foundation for Innovation in Medicine. DeFelice defined a nutraceutical as "Food, or parts of a food, that provide medical or health benefits, including the prevention and treatment of disease."[132]

Using food for both nutrition and medicinal purposes is nothing new. It has been part of many ancient cultures. In fact, the concept of nutraceuticals is nearly 3,000 years old! It began to catch on when Hippocrates, the father of modern medicine, recognized the relationship between food and health.

The people of India and China have a long tradition of eating natural foods that are known to be medicinal. Countries like Germany, France, and England were among the first to say that diet is more important than both exercise and genetic factors for people to attain good health.

Today, nutraceuticals have evolved from their traditional background to a highly scientific field where the quality, safety, and effectiveness of the products are backed by evidence, research, and state-of-the-art technology.

How Nutraceuticals Work

A healthy diet contributes to your health by providing the nutrients your body needs to repair itself, grow, and function well. When your diet does not supply enough of these essential nutrients and vitamins, or if the healthy foods you are eating are grown in depleted soils, nutraceuticals can help fill those gaps. In addition, certain health conditions, including Hashimoto's can lead to nutrient deficiencies and taking larger doses of certain nutrients can correct or improve those conditions.

As covered in Chapter 5, the most common nutrient deficiencies in people with Hashimoto's are vitamin D, vitamin B12, selenium, iron, magnesium, zinc, and thiamine (B1). This chapter describes these nutrients and several other proven nutraceuticals that help people with Hashimoto's disease and adrenal fatigue.

Selenium

Selenium is an essential trace mineral that is critical to your thyroid health. The thyroid gland has the highest concentration of selenium of any organ in the body. Selenium protects the thyroid from inflammation. It acts as an antioxidant and anti-inflammatory. Selenium is needed to produce thyroid hormone *and* to convert T4 thyroid hormone to T3 thyroid hormone (the most active form).

A selenium deficiency can cause symptoms of hypothyroidism, including extreme fatigue, mental slowness, goiter, muscle weakness, hair loss, infertility, and recurrent miscarriages.

Several studies have shown that selenium supplementation significantly reduces thyroid antibodies (TPO-Ab and Tg-Ab), which are an indicator of Hashimoto's. The higher the antibody levels were at the beginning of the studies, the more they were reduced by taking selenium.

Selenium has also been shown to reduce activity of the Epstein-Barr Virus (EBV) which is a virus linked to Hashimoto's and other autoimmune diseases. Selenium is also helpful in inhibiting other herpes viruses such as Herpes 6 which is also linked with Hashimoto's disease.

Regional Selenium Deficiency

The selenium content in foods depends on the quality of the soil used to grow them. The most selenium-deficient areas in the United States are the Northwest, Northeast, the Atlantic coastal area, Florida, and regions surrounding the Great Lakes. If you live in any of these areas, you should ensure your family supplements with selenium or eats selenium-rich foods grown in other regions to lower the risk of cancer, thyroid disease, and cardiovascular disease.

A study in China compared 6132 people from two counties, one of which had low of levels of selenium in the soil, and the other with adequate selenium in the soil. Researchers found that there was a higher incidence of thyroid conditions (hypothyroidism, subclinical hypothyroidism, autoimmune thyroiditis, and enlarged thyroid) in the low-selenium group. The people in the county with adequate selenium levels had a significantly lower risk of thyroid conditions.[133]

Selenium and Glutathione

Selenium is needed to produce glutathione. Glutathione is your body's master antioxidant and is essential to your immune system function. Glutathione plays a critical role in the body's detoxification processes. It binds to toxins and transforms them in such a way that the body can eliminate them effectively via the urine or bile. Selenium also helps to prevent damage to the liver caused by toxins and supports the liver's ability to break down and eliminate toxins.

Selenium Supplementation During Pregnancy

In Chapter 2, I described postpartum thyroiditis (PPT). This inflammatory thyroid condition can result in permanent hypothyroidism after giving birth to a child. What about preventative steps? Could selenium supplementation during pregnancy prevent thyroid inflammation?

Possibly, yes. A study published in the *Journal of Clinical Endocrinology & Metabolism* found that pregnant women who tested positive for Thyroid Peroxidase Antibodies (TPOAb) are prone to develop PPT and permanent hypothyroidism. In this study, one group of mothers received 200 mcg of selenium daily and the other group received a placebo. The results showed that selenium supplementation during pregnancy and the postpartum period reduced the incidence of hypothyroidism.[134]

Imagine if OB/GYNs in all selenium-deficient regions of the world simply advised pregnant mothers to supplement with selenium? If only this was done, perhaps a lot of needless disease could be prevented!

Recommendations

L-Selenomethionine is the preferred form of selenium because it has a superior absorption rate compared with other forms of selenium used in supplements. It is the form found naturally in food and about 90 percent of it is absorbed. 200–400 mcg is the recommended dose.

If you have Hashimoto's disease, then it is reasonable to supplement with selenomethionine, but you should consider the selenium content in foods you are eating as well as other supplements you take so you don't exceed the safe range.

Brazil nuts can contain anywhere from 0.2 mcg to 253 mcg of selenium depending on where they are grown. Thus, if you eat three Brazil nuts a day, you can avoid taking a selenium supplement. Consuming over 800 mcg of selenium per day can be toxic. The side effects of too much selenium are similar to many other conditions so it's not easy to figure out without testing. I recently asked my doctor about selenium testing and he advised me that it has to be specifically requested. It's not part of routine blood work. It would be helpful if you can determine if you have too much or too little selenium.

Magnesium

This might sound extreme, but I read an entire book about magnesium, called the *Miracle Mineral,* by Carolyn Dean M.D. N.D. I geek out on things like this because nature has so many answers for us. I was just amazed at how many functions this mineral has. It's a supplement I recommend often to people. It helps to relieve menstrual cramps, headaches, restless legs, muscle cramps, insomnia, and constipation. I personally had unbearable menstrual cramps until I started regularly supplementing with magnesium in my early twenties.

Magnesium is needed for more than 300 biochemical processes in the body. It is the fourth most abundant essential mineral in the human body after sodium, potassium, and calcium. It helps to regulate the heartbeat and blood pressure and helps to maintain normal nerve and muscle function. It helps to strengthen the bones, supports the immune system, and helps with the production of energy. Magnesium can help with exercise recovery (a common issue with Hashimoto's) because it helps move blood sugar into your muscles and dispose of lactate, which can build up during exercise and cause muscle fatigue.

Magnesium also helps to keep blood glucose levels steady. Studies found that about **48 percent of people with type 2 diabetes have low levels of magnesium.**[135] This might disrupt the body's ability to regulate blood sugar levels effectively. This is a huge finding! Nearly half of people with type 2 diabetes are struggling with low magnesium.

So, how many endocrinologists are checking the magnesium levels of their diabetes patients and recommending proper supplementation to help them with their blood sugar management? My guess is little to none.

Does magnesium directly benefit the thyroid? Yes! Some studies have shown that long-term magnesium supplementation, in addition to selenium and coenzyme Q10, helps to:

- Lower thyroid antibodies
- Improve the appearance of the thyroid gland on ultrasound tests
- Reduce the occurrence of thyroid and breast nodules[136]

These are three distinct thyroid benefits for those of us struggling to manage Hashimoto's disease! Magnesium is a MUST!

There are many magnesium supplements to choose from and at least eight different types of magnesium, and they serve different purposes. For example, magnesium citrate is commonly used to relieve constipation. Magnesium L-threonate is helpful to the nervous system as it is the only form of magnesium known to cross the blood-brain barrier. There are a lot of magnesium formulas to choose from and plenty of information online. Many sites, however, do not mention magnesium L-threonate, which is a superior form for people experiencing neurological conditions or issues with anxiety, depression, memory, or concentration.

Recommendations

- It's better to take a formula with multiple forms of magnesium because they act in different ways and provide multiple benefits to the body.
- Take a magnesium complex in the morning to support your brain function and stress response throughout the day.
- Take magnesium L-threonate (or a magnesium complex) in the evening to promote relaxation and neurological health.
- It is better to take magnesium on an empty stomach to absorb it more efficiently, however, if your stomach gets upset, take it with a small amount of food.

Vitamin B1 (Thiamine)

Thiamine deficiency is linked to chronic fatigue but rarely shows up as a deficiency on lab work. Thiamine is one of the B vitamins, vitamin B1. Its main function is to change carbohydrates into energy. Thiamine is needed to release the appropriate amount of hydrochloric acid into the stomach to help digest proteins and fats. Many people with Hashimoto's have low stomach acid and sometimes experience digestive problems. This can impede the absorption of nutrients.

The recommended daily allowance for thiamine is 1.1 mg for women above 19 years old but for several reasons, this small amount is not enough for those with autoimmune thyroid disease.

One reason to supplement with B1 is because many dietary sources of B1 (fortified grains, bread, cereal, eggs, beef liver, pork, legumes, dried milk, peas, nuts, and seeds) are avoided on grain-free diets. Other than liver and pork, **most foods containing B1 are restricted on the Paleo diet,** and **all of them are restricted on the Autoimmune Paleo** diet. In addition, stress can cause B vitamins to be depleted.

Thiamine deficiency is rare and usually found in alcoholics, but is also found in people that have Hashimoto's, Crohn's, or other autoimmune conditions, irritable bowel syndrome (IBS), fatigue, low blood pressure, low stomach acid, anorexia, brain fog, or adrenal issues. Some medications can also deplete the body of thiamine.

Symptoms of a mild thiamine deficiency include depression, irritability, fatigue, low blood pressure, abdominal discomfort, and trouble digesting carbohydrates.

Italian clinicians Dr. Antonio Costantini and nurse Maria Immacolata Pala hypothesized that a mild thiamine deficiency might cause the chronic fatigue that affects people with inflammatory and autoimmune diseases. They conducted the following two studies to test this hypothesis.

- In a study of people with ulcerative colitis and Crohn's disease, all 12 patients suffered chronic fatigue. Their blood tests for thiamine were normal, but researchers suspected that thiamine was not being transported to cells like it should be. After being given high doses of thiamine (600 mg), the fatigue was completely resolved in 10 of the 12 people, and partially resolved in the other two people.[137]
- After the researchers found that thiamine helped relieve fatigue in people with ulcerative colitis, they conducted another study of three women with Hashimoto's who were on Levothyroxin thyroid medication yet still suffered chronic fatigue. Two of the women took an oral dose of thiamine (600 mg) each day, while the third was given an injection of 100 mg, every four days. Two of the women had complete remission of their fatigue and the third had a significant improvement. **The woman who was given a thiamine injection felt her fatigue lift within six hours. The women who took oral doses of thiamine felt better within three to five days.**[138]

What does this mean? The blood work for these folks did *not* reveal a thiamine deficiency, yet high-dose supplementation of thiamine resolved their fatigue. This means that fatigue is caused by a mild thiamine deficiency that is not detected with blood work in people with autoimmune disease.

The researchers explained that it is likely due to a problem with the transport of thiamine inside the cells, which is likely to be related to the autoimmune process of the disease. They concluded that taking large doses of thiamine can restore processes in the body that need thiamine, including fatigue.

How would you ever discover this? I have never discussed thiamine with any of my doctors. I learned about this from the Thyroid

Pharmacist, Dr. Izabella Wentz. In fact, Dr. Wentz surveyed 2,232 people with Hashimoto's disease and found that 36 percent of them reported that B1 supplementation made them feel better.

Recommendations

Dr. Wentz recommends taking benfotiamine, rather than other forms of thiamine. Benfotiamine is similar to thiamine (vitamin B1) but is better absorbed. Potential benefits include an increase in energy and brain function, and improved blood pressure and blood sugar balance. I recommend working with a functional medicine physician to determine your dose. You may need higher doses initially if you are fatigued and then lower periodic doses after you regain your energy.

Vitamin B12

Vitamin B12 is a water-soluble vitamin that is needed for growth, protein synthesis, cognitive function, and cell reproduction. Foods that are rich in B12 include meat, fish, eggs, and dairy products.

B12 deficiency can cause many symptoms some of which include depression, fatigue, cognitive problems, feeling of pins and needles, weakness, palpitations, lack of appetite, and impaired digestion. Cracks in the corners of the mouth are also a symptom that is more commonly experienced in the elderly.

The following are some of the factors that can lead to a B12 deficiency:

- Hypothyroidism inhibits absorption of nutrients from the food you eat
- Having low stomach acid can prevent you from absorbing the B12 in foods you eat
- Some medications alter your gut flora and deplete nutrients (such as antibiotics, birth control, and acid reflux medications)
- Following a diet with little to no meat, fish, and dairy foods

- Small intestinal bacterial overgrowth (SIBO) causes decreased absorption of B12

B12 is a water-soluble vitamin, which means that it doesn't get stored in fat, and it is eliminated quickly if it is not used by the body.

In contrast, if your B12 result is elevated, it can be due to an MTHFR gene variation. People with MTHFR gene variations might not be able to properly use non-methylated B12 (such as the B12 in the foods they eat). In this case, they may have elevated levels of B12 on lab work, but they will have low levels of the type of B12 that their body can utilize. This was the case with me. My B12 lab results were very high. No doctor ever explained to me why. So, I didn't think I needed supplementation. Now, I take sublingual B12 (methylcobalamin) to ensure I get enough. I take 3,000 mcg almost every day. My recent B12 lab result was normal.

Recommendations

Vitamin B12 blood tests usually have a normal range between 200–900 pg/mL. A B12 result less than 200 pg/mL indicates a deficiency.

If you have a B12 deficiency, you can take sublingual doses of 5 mg (5000 mcg) of methylated B12, daily for several weeks to correct the deficiency and afterwards take a maintenance dose of 1,500–3,000 mcg and try to eat foods rich in vitamin B12.

Zinc

Optimizing your zinc level may help reduce your symptoms of Hashimoto's. Zinc is an essential trace element found in foods such as beef, chicken, pork, lobster, and oysters. The body cannot make it on its own, but small amounts are important to our health. Zinc acts as a catalyst for hundreds of bodily functions. You need adequate zinc for a healthy sense of taste and smell, detoxification, gut health, immune function, wound healing, converting T4 to T3, and the production of TSH.

Zinc can help heal and seal the intestinal junctions of people with intestinal permeability. Healthy levels of zinc can help fight viral infections and colds by balancing the immune system's response. If you are very low in zinc, this prevents your body from converting T4 hormone into the active T3 version. This could lead to problems such as fatigue, weight gain, brittle nails, and hair loss, *even if* you are taking a thyroid medication such as levothyroxine.

A study of overweight female hypothyroid patients in 2015 found that taking zinc alone or in combination with selenium, has a positive effect on thyroid function. The women received either a zinc supplement, a selenium supplement, placebo pills, or a combination of both zinc and selenium supplements. After three months, the group taking the zinc and selenium combination, and the group taking only zinc, had a significant increase in their free T3 levels. The group that took both zinc and selenium had a significant decrease in their TSH and an increase in T4 levels.[139]

Recommendations

Zinc picolinate has a better absorption rate than other forms of zinc. Do not take more than 30 mg daily unless advised by your doctor. Take it with food to avoid nausea and take it at least two hours away from iron supplements for better absorption.

Iron (Ferritin)

Hashimoto's patients are often deficient in iron because malabsorption of nutrients is a common problem in people with autoimmune thyroid disease. It's important to know your iron status. On your lab work, it will be listed as "ferritin." Your ferritin level should be above 50 ng/mL. A deficiency in iron (including the more severe form called anemia) can significantly affect your thyroid function and negatively impact your treatment.

Low levels of iron can lead to fatigue, difficulty breathing, and hair loss. Women who are menstruating or are postpartum may be at increased risk of low iron due to blood loss. Health conditions that affect our gut microbiota can also cause a ferritin deficiency. Vegan or vegetarian diets and heavy metal toxicity are also factors related to low ferritin levels.

Foods that contain iron include meat, poultry, eggs, organ meats, pumpkin seeds, chickpeas, and lentils.

Recommendations

If you are iron deficient and need to supplement, you should work with your health practitioner to determine the best dosage and form of ferritin to use.

Alternatively, if you have too much iron in your body, it can be toxic. You can lower excess levels of iron by donating blood. You can also consume beverages (such as cocoa or black or green tea) and foods that block iron absorption.

Vitamin D3 and Vitamin K2

Vitamin D is an important part of a healthy life for everyone, but extra important for people with cancer, thyroid disease, and autoimmune disease. It is an essential nutrient and a hormone that plays an important role for many processes within the body. Vitamin D is produced in the skin when exposed to sunlight. Vitamin D is also found in certain foods, such as fatty fish and fortified dairy products but *only* about 10 percent of vitamin D is absorbed through the diet. The liver and kidneys convert vitamin D into the active hormone, which is called calcitriol (2.25-dihydroxyvitamin D).

Most people are familiar with its bone strengthening benefits, but vitamin D is an unsung hero. It has benefits for every system of the body. Vitamin D has been shown to reduce cancer cell growth, help control infections, reduce inflammation, and reduce the risk of depression, dementia, heart disease, and stroke. It also helps to **prevent and modulate autoimmune disease**.

One of the most important and powerful functions of vitamin D is how it helps us to fight pathogens. There are vitamin D receptors and activating enzymes on *every* surface of *every* white blood cell. When your body has enough vitamin D, the pathogen-fighting effects of your monocytes and macrophages are stronger. These are special white blood cells that help decrease inflammation and defend you from infections, viruses, the flu, and even cancer! Vitamin D expert, Dr. William Grant, Ph.D., indicated that if the optimal serum vitamin D level were raised, it would prevent **30 percent of cancer deaths annually.**

It is of utmost importance if you have autoimmune disease to "know your number" and try to keep your vitamin D level on the high end of the range. It is considered a vitamin D deficiency if you have a blood level of 25-hydroxyvitamin (25 OH D) of less than 30 ng/mL The Endocrine Society recommends a range of 40–60 ng/mL.[140] However, functional medicine doctors and many holistic experts recommend a range from **50–80 ng/ mL** for optimal effect and for management of autoimmune disease.

Challenges to Absorption of Vitamin D

There are several factors that affect your ability to absorb vitamin D. It is not as simple as just getting some sun. Even people that live in sunny climates have deficient vitamin D levels. To absorb a significant amount of vitamin D from the sun, you must have at least 50–75 percent of your skin exposed. Other factors to consider include the UV index and time of day. Your body's ability to absorb and utilize vitamin D is another factor. Absorbing vitamin D from the sun is more difficult for people with obesity, diabetes, thicker skin, or thicker pigment. It's also harder for people with a fatty liver or gallbladder issues because bile is needed to absorb vitamin D.

Testing for Deficiency

How do you know if you are deficient? Many people don't know they are vitamin D deficient because there are no obvious symptoms. Some common signs of a vitamin D deficiency can mimic other conditions, such as fatigue and depression. Some of these symptoms are not experienced for months or even years after you become deficient. The best way to know for sure is to ask your doctor for a vitamin D test.

It was almost 10 years after having symptoms of thyroid disease that a doctor finally ran a vitamin D test for me. I visited an integrative MD that trained with the American College for Advancement in Medicine (ACAM).[141] My first vitamin D blood test result was 40 ng/mL. The range for the test was 30–100 ng/mL so at 40, I was in range but on the low end. I had been taking a 2,000 IU vitamin D3 supplement prior to testing, so my level may have been lower previously. That doctor recommended that I take 10,000 IU daily, which I did. After a year, my level went up to 60. I felt a huge difference. I felt less depressed and anxious. I stopped getting the flu and bronchitis every year. I may also have stronger bones because I haven't suffered any more sprained ankles. I used to sprain an ankle almost every spring when I started working out trying to get in shape for summer!

Is 10,000 UI too much? No! It is not even 1 milligram. It's 0.25 mg, or 250 micrograms. Is there a risk of taking that much? No. On the contrary, there is a risk of **not** taking that much. Some doctors prescribe 50,000 IU and more depending on the patient. In the United States, approximately 42 percent of adults are vitamin D deficient, while 50 percent of children between age one to five, and 70 percent of children between age six to eleven have low vitamin D levels. The statistics are different for people with dark skin. Nearly 63 percent of Hispanic adults and 82 percent of African American adults are vitamin D deficient.[142]

The RDA is 600–800 IU and this is based on old research about preventing rickets or osteoporosis. It does not account for updated research about its preventative effects for many diseases including autoimmune disease, cancer, depression, heart disease, dementia, and more.

The Calcium and Vitamin K Connection

Many people with autoimmune disease eliminate or reduce grains in their diet. Dr. William Davis, cardiologist and author of *Wheat Belly, Super Gut,* and *Undoctored,* recommends a grain-free diet, vitamin D, and magnesium for bone health. However, he warns that **when you reduce or eliminate grains, you may have increased calcium absorption in your intestines and less calcium excreted in urine.** If you have too much calcium in your blood, this is called hypercalcemia, and this condition has been shown to weaken bones, create **kidney stones,** and interfere with normal functioning of your heart and brain. In this case, you should *avoid* calcium supplements because of the increased calcium absorption that is caused by eliminating grains from your diet.

To help your body use calcium correctly, it is important that you get enough vitamin K1 and K2. Vitamin K1 is found in green vegetables. Vitamin K2 is found in chicken, beef liver, egg yolks, butter (from grass-fed animals only), and fermented foods, such as cheeses, sauerkraut, and fermented soybean products such as natto. K1 participates in blood coagulation. K1 and K2 deficiency can lead to loss of bone calcium which leads to osteoporosis, hip fractures, and other fractures.

It can also result in calcium building up in your arteries, which can cause atherosclerosis and lead to heart attacks. Lack of K2 can also result in tartar buildup on the teeth and the hardening of body tissues that causes arthritis, bursitis, reduced flexibility, stiffness, and pain.

A small amount of K2 is produced in the body by a bacterial conversion process when K1 gets converted to K2 in the intestines. It has been suggested that this conversion may be negatively impacted if you have a gut imbalance. In that case, taking a K2 supplement can help build bone density and reduce cardiovascular risk.

Recommendations

Get plenty of vitamin D from sunlight, fermented cod liver oil, or a vitamin D3 supplement. Vitamin D3 is the correct form to supplement with, not D2. It typically comes in gel caps, but also comes in liquid form. I prefer and recommend 5,000 IU gel caps with olive oil, not soybean oil. Your dose is dependent on your current vitamin D level and on your ability to absorb vitamin D. Gel caps work well for me, but some people prefer liquid vitamin D products. Either are fine.

Try to get vitamin K1 by consuming four to five servings daily of green vegetables and K2 by consuming foods rich in K2. You can also choose to take a vitamin K supplement or a combination vitamin D3 and K2 supplement.

Don't forget that exercising is a must to increase bone density, especially weight-bearing exercises. Exercise that involves impact to the spine, such as jogging, jumping rope, stair climbing, hopping in place, and dancing, helps to increase bone density. Simply jumping in place 10 to 20 times or taking a 20-minute walk daily can provide significant measurable increases in bone density.

Medicinal Mushrooms

Mushrooms are an incredible source of medicine. The healing and immune-stimulating properties of mushrooms have been known for thousands of years in Eastern countries.

Medicinal mushrooms are immune modulators. What is immunomodulation? It is the automatic adjustment of the immune system to maintain a balanced immune response. Essentially, they help to calm your immune system down when it's overactive or boost it when needed to fight. Medicinal mushrooms are also used to prevent and treat cancer.

David "Avocado" Wolfe, internationally renowned health expert, author, farmer, and avid mushroom hunter, teaches a course about medicinal mushrooms in his Nutrition Certification program (which I completed in 2016). When David talks about mushrooms, I listen. He says that reishi and chaga are considered the king and queen of the mushroom kingdom. They both have tremendous health benefits many of which are described in this section.

Some people are concerned about poisonous mushrooms. David explains that most poisonous mushrooms grow on the ground, NOT on trees. Most medicinal mushrooms studied and recommended are **tree** mushrooms. There is only one tree mushroom that is toxic—the "Jack O'Lantern" mushroom, and it's very rare and glows in the dark. In fact, in all of David's mushroom hunting journeys, he has never encountered one!

Although medicinal mushrooms can be eaten, you can take medicinal doses of them in supplement form. They come in liquid extracts, capsules, powders, or whole dried chunks.

Benefits of Medicinal Mushrooms

Medicinal mushrooms are nutritional powerhouses with many proven health benefits. They help to modulate the immune system which is important for people with Hashimoto's and other autoimmune diseases. They also help to support the nervous system with mood and brain health.

Asian cultures have used certain mushrooms for centuries as a natural cancer treatment. Medicinal mushrooms lower cancer risk in several ways. They supply germanium, a nutrient that boosts oxygen use in the body and fights free radical damage. In fact, in traditional Chinese medicine, over 200 mushroom species are used and 25 percent of those are found to effectively fight harmful tumors.

Mushrooms are also excellent sources of **antioxidants** as they contain polyphenols and selenium, which are common in the plant world. But they also contain antioxidants that are unique to mushrooms. One of these special antioxidants is ergothioneine, which scientists recognize as a master antioxidant. A study in the journal *Nature* described ergothioneine as "an unusual sulfur-containing derivative of the amino acid, histidine." It plays a role in protecting your DNA from oxidative damage. This means that **mushrooms protect your DNA**. Several types of DNA damage in humans occurs either naturally or from environmental factors. This DNA damage is distinctly different from genetic mutations, although both are types of errors in DNA.

Mushrooms are also rich in **polyphenols** which give fruits, berries, and vegetables their vibrant colors. Polyphenols have the following benefits:

- Fight cancer cells and inhibit angiogenesis (the growth of blood vessels that feed a tumor)
- Protect your skin against ultraviolet radiation
- Reduce inflammation
- Protect your cardiovascular system
- Promote normal blood pressure
- Neutralize free radicals
- Reduce the appearance of aging
- Promote brain health, and protect against dementia
- Support normal blood sugar levels

Mushroom expert Paul Stamets shared that humans share close to 50 percent of their DNA with fungi, and we get many of the same viruses as fungi. Stamet said, "If we can identify the natural immunities that fungi have developed, we can extract them to help humans."[143] There is a lot of research going on in this area. We may soon have antiviral drugs made from fungi.

According to Riikka Linnakoski, a forest pathologist at the Natural Resources Institute, Finland, compounds produced by fungi have already been identified that can destroy viruses that cause diseases such as mumps, measles, flu, polio, and glandular fever. Several fungi have also been shown to produce compounds that could potentially treat "incurable" diseases such as HIV and the Zika virus.[144] This could be helpful in treating some of the root causes that trigger autoimmune disease. In the meantime, supplementing with the medicinal mushrooms described in this section is a safe and natural way to improve your health and prevent disease.

Reishi

Ganoderma lucidum, known as reishi in Japan and lingzhi in China, is referred to as the "Mushroom of Immortality". It has been extensively studied for its many health-enhancing properties and benefits. It has been used in traditional Chinese medicine for over 2000 years for many conditions, including overall health and longevity.[145] Over the last three decades, medicinal mushrooms such as reishi, chaga, and turkey tail have been used in Japan, China, and Korea for the prevention and treatment of cancer as well as treatment for chemotherapy side effects.[146]

Reishi is an adaptogenic herb. It doesn't stimulate the thyroid, liver, kidney, or your overall system. It *regulates* them. It does not stimulate or suppress the immune system. It is an **immune modulator**.

Although many mushrooms have immune boosting properties, red reishi has the longest history of successful use in treating the widest range of health problems. Compared to other mushrooms, only reishi has **terpenes**, which are the main group of compounds responsible for its many health benefits. The terpenes make the reishi bitter in taste and strong in aroma. In fact, terpenes are key to creating many essential oils. Essential oils high in terpenes include anise, oregano, citrus, cinnamon, pine, and clove, among others. Terpenes are considered the strongest anti-inflammatory and anti-tumor compounds found in nature. If that is not incredible enough, one of the most useful properties of terpenes is their ability to dissolve, dissipate, and decompose cellular matter. As mentioned in Chapter 9, reishi is one of the best plants in the world for flushing out cellular waste from your body, so it is an excellent tool to use when detoxing and **reducing your viral load**!

Reishi also helps with **metabolism** by improving insulin resistance. In studies, a reishi compound reduced weight, increased insulin levels, and reduced blood glucose with an effect comparable to the drug Metformin! It also improved blood levels of triglycerides, total cholesterol, low-density lipoprotein cholesterol (LDL-C), and high-density lipoprotein cholesterol (HDL-C).[147]

Additional proven benefits of reishi include:

- Helps with lung cancer, leukemia, and other cancers
- Antibacterial, antiviral (herpes, Epstein-Barr), antifungal (including candida)
- Anti-inflammatory
- Helps reduce symptoms of rheumatoid arthritis
- Supports liver, digestion, and glycemic balance
- Helps lower blood pressure
- Reduces anxiety and depression
- Protects your DNA

Reishi is useful for many ailments. It has immunostimulant properties, calms anxiety, and is used as a general tonic. It is antiallergenic and antiviral and is used for hepatitis and heart arrhythmias. Hobbs writes that this mushroom is "especially suitable as a **calming herb for people with anxiety, sleeplessness, or nervousness accompanied by an adrenal weakness.**"

David Wolfe said, "Reishi taken long term imparts a *sense of calm*".

Chaga

Chaga mushroom, known as Inonotus obliquus, is known as the king of the mushroom kingdom because it has many impressive and powerful health benefits. Chaga grows on mature live birch trees in the northern hemisphere. It is nicknamed the diamond of the forest, but it doesn't look like a diamond! It's black and brown and looks like burned charcoal but if you look inside, you will find a nutrient-rich, rusty, yellowish-brown interior. It's consumed mostly as a tea, but also in coffee. It can also be taken as a liquid tincture or in capsule form.

It is one of the most powerful antioxidants in the world. The Oxygen Radical Absorbency Capacity or ORAC score measures the antioxidant strength of foods. Chaga's **ORAC score is 146,700.**[249] Its antioxidant level is 1,300 times that of blueberries and 80 times that of pomegranates.

Chaga has over 200 different compounds, including polysaccharides, beta-glucans, melanins, and polyphenols. It also contains vitamin D, vitamin B, amino acids, iron, potassium, calcium, magnesium, selenium, and zinc. It's also high in germanium which is antiviral.

The most well-known benefits of chaga include:

- Fights all types of cancer
- Blood sugar regulation
- Improves the health of the skin, liver, and stomach
- Supports heart health
- Supports healthy cholesterol levels
- Increases energy, stamina, and endurance
- Helps immune system to fight bacterial and viral infections

Most impressive are its anticancer benefits. David Wolfe, author of *Chaga: King of the Medicinal Mushrooms* said, "Chaga is the most powerful cancer-fighting herb known and fights all kinds of radiation damage to healthy tissue."

Laboratory mice given chaga experienced a 60 percent reduction in tumors.[148] A study published in the *World Journal of Gastroenterology* found that chaga prevents the growth of cancerous liver cells.[149] In 2021, a review of both recent and prior research was published regarding chaga mushroom benefits. It has been used in Kiev to cure lip tumors for centuries. It has been found to cause the death of multiple types of cancer cells, including liver, lung, ovarian, and cervical.[150]

Chaga mushrooms contains beta glucans, which are biologically active polysaccharides that exist in many mushrooms and other plants. These are well-known and well-researched compounds that have therapeutic properties against metabolic syndrome, obesity, diabetes, hypercholesterolemia (high LDL), and hypertension.[151] Chaga has been shown to increase good cholesterol (HDL) and lower bad cholesterol (LDL) and triglycerides. Beta-glucans also reduce the spread of tumors and prevent metastasis.[152]

One of the most unusual but incredible impactful benefits of chaga is its success in healing psoriasis. In several Russian studies, the majority of psoriasis patients who took chaga recovered completely from their psoriasis.

Caution: If you have an oxalate build-up, chaga is not for you. Chaga mushrooms are high in oxalates. Excessive intake could cause problems if you already have oxalate build-up.

Turkey Tail

The Trametes versicolor mushroom, known as turkey tail, is beautiful. It grows in the northern forests of the world and is named for its colorful wavy stripes, some blue and some brown. It is known for having strong antiviral, antimicrobial, and antitumor properties. These properties have been attributed to two polysaccharides, polysaccharide-K (PSK), also known as krestin, and polysaccharide-P (PSP).

The Japanese government approved the use of PSK in the 1980s for treating several types of cancers. It is currently used in Japan together with surgery, chemotherapy, and radiation. In Japanese trials, PSK was shown to extend survival by five years or more in patients with cancers of the stomach, colon/rectum, esophagus, nasopharynx, and lung (non-small cell types).

Benefits of turkey tail include:

- Supports immune health
- Boosts immunity in cancer patients
- Lessens side effects of chemotherapy
- Supports normal cellular growth
- Aids respiratory health
- Support urinary and digestive health
- Anticancer
- Antiviral

Cordyceps

This unique mushroom has a long history of providing benefits to the immune system, respiratory health, vital energy, and more. In fact, Chinese emperors in the past used this mushroom exclusively, thus perpetuating the phrase, "Ancient Chinese Secret!"

Once available to the public, and out of the greedy emperors' hands, traditional healers suggested it for "all illnesses" as a general tonic, because they observed that it improved energy, appetite, stamina, endurance, libido, and sleep.

Benefits of cordyceps include:

- Immune modulator
- Anti-tumor
- Anti-microbial
- Antiviral
- Anti-inflammatory
- Asthma support
- Rheumatoid arthritis relief
- Kidney support
- Stroke recovery
- Stamina for athletes and harsh climates

Lion's Mane

Lion's mane mushrooms, also known as hericium erinaceus, are easy to identify. They have a unique white shaggy appearance, resembling a lion's mane. They are delicious to eat but their real value comes from their medicinal benefits. They are most widely known for their cognitive and neurological benefits. Some of the compounds extracted from lion's mane have been shown to help people recover from (or at least improve) brain conditions including depression, Alzheimer's disease, Parkinson's disease, and spinal cord injury.[153] Lion's mane has been used traditionally in Chinese medicine to treat stomach problems. It helps to treat h. Pylori,[154] ulcers,[155] colitis, and inflammatory bowel disease (IBD).[156]

One of the most exciting and impressive benefits of lion's mane is its ability to repair nerve damage. I've heard many people say that nerve damage cannot be repaired, but lion's mane has been shown to help to repair damaged nerves. A study published in 2012 by the *International Journal of Medicinal Mushrooms* studied the effects of lion's mane mushroom on nerve repair and reached an impressive conclusion. Specifically, they found that daily oral supplementation of lion's mane promoted the regeneration of injured peroneal nerves in rats during the early stages of recovery.[157]

Lion's mane has a compound called hericenones, which helps to promote Nerve Growth Factor (NGF) in the body. NGF is known for helping to support the growth and survival of nerve cells in the brain as well as other areas. NGF has been found to help with motor function, the growth of nerve tissue, regulation of the immune system, and the survival of pancreatic (insulin-producing) beta cells.

Additional benefits include the following:

- Provides neuroprotection
- May help stroke recovery
- Anticancer
- Powerful antioxidant
- Helps with depression, anxiety, and insomnia
- Enhances memory and brain function
- Helps to reduce blood sugar and associated excessive thirst[158]
- Helps with Alzheimer's disease[159]

Agaricus Blazei

Agaricus blazei is another edible mushroom that is also medicinal. It is also known as the sun mushroom in Brazil and the royal sun mushroom in other countries. It's one of the highest protein sources in the mushroom kingdom and contain many nutrients including enzymes, bioactive compounds, amino acids, antioxidants, phosphorus, iron, calcium, vitamin B1, B2, niacin, and the antioxidant ergosterol.

Agaricus blazei has strong anti-tumor[248], anti-inflammatory, and anti-allergic effects.[160] Research has shown that it has significant effects on sarcoma, lung, breast, and ovarian cancers. Agaricus blazei has also shown impressive results in studies for people with diabetes type 2, including improvements in insulin resistance, hyperglycemia, cholesterol levels, and arterial plaque buildup.[161]

Shitake

Shitake is the second most popular edible mushroom in the world. It is widely known for its health benefits. Shitake is rich in B vitamins. Shitake is anticancer, anti-fungal, antiviral, antibacterial, and anti-candida. It lowers blood pressure and cholesterol and prevents atherosclerosis. Shitake improves immunity, kills selective skin cancer cells without harming normal cells, and inhibits growth of breast tumor cells. It also protects the liver against damage from the pain reliever acetaminophen.

Maitake

Maitake are edible mushrooms that have been known to grow to over 100 pounds! Maitake is an adaptogen, and thus supports autoimmune conditions. Maitake also has strong anti-diabetic properties. Maitake is also anticancer, lowers blood pressure, and supports cardiovascular health and metabolic balance.

Recommendations

Dosages vary depending on which mushrooms you take, and which conditions you want to address. I suggest you follow the instructions on the product label. For overall immunity and wellness, you can choose a product with a blend. Mushrooms that help to modulate autoimmune conditions include reishi, chaga, cordyceps, maitake, turkey tail, and agaricus blazei. I prefer reputable brands that grow the mushrooms organically in greenhouses in the US.

I personally take reishi, chaga, agaricus, and lion's mane regularly and sometimes use blends. I use liquid tinctures, capsules, and powder products.

Myo & D-Chiro Inositol

Myo & D-chiro inositol supplements have proven benefits for thyroid disease, polycystic ovary syndrome (PCOS), metabolic syndrome (insulin resistance), and diabetes type 2. Multiple studies have shown that Hashimoto's patients treated with both myo-inositol and selenium experienced reductions in TPOAb thyroid antibodies and TSH levels, restoring *euthyroidism*, which means normal thyroid function.[162][163]

Inositol is a type of sugar alcohol, that is produced in our bodies and found in foods such as fruits, beans, and nuts. Myo-inositol and D-chiro inositol are two out of nine forms of inositol that are commonly taken as supplements and are studied as a combination treatment. Myo-inositol has antioxidant, anti-diabetic, anti-inflammatory, and anticancer properties. People with Hashimoto's can be deficient in inositol due to poor nutrient absorption, high glucose levels, or genetic reasons.[164]

Myo & D-chiro inositol can help lower glucose levels after a meal and can also help with diabetic neuropathy. For women with PCOS (polycystic ovary syndrome), it can help regulate menstrual cycles, improve insulin sensitivity, decrease insulin and androgen levels, and reduce hirsutism and acne.[165]

Myo-inositol is also an effective treatment for postmenopausal women with metabolic syndrome. One study found that after six months of taking myo-inositol, postmenopausal women with metabolic syndrome had improvements in blood pressure, cholesterol (triglycerides and HDL), and insulin resistance.[166]

Recommendations

I recommend taking a Myo & D-chiro inositol supplement as directed on the label with selenium. These supplements may take a month or two to show effects.

Adrenal Support Herbs

As mentioned in Chapter 5, adrenal fatigue affects our energy, weight, mood, sleep, and more. Cortisol is excreted by your adrenal glands when you experience stress. Many people with Hashimoto's have low cortisol levels. If you experience the symptoms of adrenal fatigue, it would be wise to support your adrenal glands.

To help your adrenals function better, you must get restorative rest, balance your blood sugar, reduce stress, lower inflammation, replenish nutrient levels, and build resilience and strength with quality supplements. It sounds like a tall order, I know. But feeling that zoom in your energy and feeling calm and happy makes it well worth the effort!

The following herbs nourish and support your adrenal glands. After replenishing and supporting your adrenals, you may feel lighter, more calm, relaxed, and positive. You may also experience better sleep and increased energy and stamina when performing your daily activities or exercising. Drink teas and/or take supplement formulas that include these herbs.

- Tulsi (Holy Basil): Tulsi is one of the most clinically proven and beneficial herbs in the world. It supports the thyroid and adrenal glands and helps the body to adapt to stress.
- Ashwagandha: Clinically proven to lower cortisol levels and inflammation. Reduces stress and anxiety, and improves blood sugar levels, mood, and memory.
- Astragalus root: Eases symptoms of adrenal fatigue. Protects against metabolic syndrome by making cells more receptive to insulin.
- Wood betony herb: Relieves stress, improves sleep quality, helps digestion, and lifts mood. Wood betony can lower blood pressure so those with low blood pressure should take caution or avoid this herb.
- Ginkgo biloba: Protects adrenal glands from free radical damage. Benefits circulation and heart health. Counteractive effect on adrenaline which reduces stress.
- Gotu kola: Eases insomnia, boosts brainpower and memory, and helps relieve depression and anxiety.

- Rhodiola rosea: Helps lower cortisol, improves sleep, combats depression, helps brain function and memory, and reduces fatigue.
- Licorice root (glycyrrhizic acid): One of the best natural remedies for the adrenals. Balances hormones and cortisol, lowers inflammation, and helps mood and stress levels.
- Lavender flower: Calms anxiety and restlessness, eases nerves, and aids sleep.
- Spearmint leaf: Reduces fatigue and stress.
- Eleuthera (Siberian ginseng) root: Improves the health of your adrenal system, which manages your body's response to stress, prevents fatigue, improve mental performance and memory.
- American ginseng: This is an adaptogenic herb with antioxidant properties that helps with physical and emotional stress and alleviates exhaustion and fatigue.
- Passionflower leaf: Increases the effects of GABA*, reduces anxiety, induces sleep, inhibits increased heart rate, high breathing rate, and racing thoughts caused by elevated levels of epinephrine and norepinephrine.

*Gamma-aminobutyric acid (GABA) is an inhibitory neurotransmitter made in the brain that affects mood and health. GABA calms your nervous system down and helps your body to react to feelings of fear, anxiety, depression, and stress.

Recommendations

Take a quality adrenal support formula with some of the ingredients listed above (take as directed on label). Tulsi, passionflower, and lavender are helpful to take before bedtime. Any form of ginseng or gotu kola are best taken in the morning as they may have a stimulating effect.

Tulsi (Holy Basil)

Tulsi is one of the greatest herbs in the world. It's been used for more than 3,000 years. It's been proven in history and in medical studies. Tulsi is an adaptogen. It helps to address physical, chemical, metabolic, and psychological stress through a unique combination of methods. One of the most well-researched abilities of this herb is keeping hormone levels balanced naturally and helping to manage anxiety. It supports thyroid and adrenal function, helps skin health, treats migraines, and protects against viruses and bacteria.

Tulsi has also been shown to prevent some cancers due to phytochemicals (such as eugenol, rosmarinic acid, apigenin, and luteolin). It prevents blood vessel growth from contributing to cancer cell growth which helps prevent metastasis.[167]

Recommendations

- Drink tulsi tea, two cups per day, one in morning and one in afternoon.
- Take in supplement form—capsules or liquid tincture.
- As an essential oil, you can rub a few drops onto your neck a few times per day or put some in a diffuser and take several deep breaths.

Ashwagandha

Ashwagandha is a well-known adaptogenic herb with a long history. Ashwagandha, also known as Indian ginseng, has been used in Ayurvedic medicine for more than 2,500 years for a wide variety of health conditions. Adaptogens help to balance your body, and ashwagandha has been shown to support adrenal health by lowering cortisol and stimulating T4 production in people with a sluggish thyroid. It also helps with thyroid hormone balance, mood, sleep, and hot flashes from menopause.

Recommendations

Take in supplement form—capsules or liquid tincture. The recommended dosage for ashwagandha varies depending on your condition. However, most benefits are associated with dosages of 225–600 mg daily for one to two months.

Turmeric, Curcumin and Tetrahydrocurcumin

Turmeric and curcumin are well known for their anti-inflammatory effects and for joint relief. Curcumin is a compound found in turmeric that has been shown to have antioxidant and anticancer properties. Turmeric and curcumin both have potential to help fight autoimmune conditions like Hashimoto's disease.

Tetrahydrocurcumin (THC) is less known but an exciting new development. THC is more bioavailable and thus more effective than turmeric and curcumin. It is a "metabolite" of curcumin. Curcumin is converted into THC (and Dihydrocurcumin (DHC)) in the liver, kidneys, and intestines. If your system doesn't convert the curcumin effectively, it may not be very bioavailable to your tissues. THC, however, is superior to curcumin in its chemical stability, bioavailability, and antioxidant activity. Both THC and DHC studies are ongoing, and they are very promising.

In a 2014 study of cadmium-toxic mice, THC reduced cadmium levels in the blood and tissues. It also helped to reverse the cadmium toxicity effects, which included hypertension, arterial stiffness, and other effects caused by severely elevated blood pressure.[168] In a 2015 study of arsenic-toxic rats, tetrahydrocurcumin significantly reduced the concentration of arsenic. It also resulted in cellular improvements to the liver tissue.[169]

Recommendations

If you choose to take a curcumin or tetrahydrocurcumin supplement, take as directed on the label or as advised by your physician. Of course, you can enjoy plenty of turmeric in your diet as well but for significant health benefits, you need a medicinal dose, and your body needs to absorb it effectively.

Berberine

Berberine is an alkaloid found in several herbs, including goldenseal, barberry, goldthread, Oregon grape, and tree turmeric. It has a deep yellow color, which indicates that it is good for the liver and digestive system. Berberine has many metabolic and cardiovascular benefits. It has been used for centuries in Asia to treat diabetes.

In 2021, a meta-analysis on berberine was performed in which 46 trials were assessed. Berberine was found to dramatically decrease A1C, insulin resistance, triglycerides, and inflammation in patients with type 2 diabetes.[170] Berberine also helps to prevent atherosclerosis, type 2 diabetes, insulin resistance, obesity, cardiovascular complications, and cancer. Berberine is one of few compounds that can activate adenosine monophosphate-activated protein kinase (AMPK), an enzyme often referred to as a "metabolic master switch." AMPK boosts fat burning which may help stop fat accumulation and protect against metabolic syndrome. [171]

Recommendations

Berberine comes in capsules, typically 500 mg per capsule. It is recommended to space out doses because berberine doesn't stay in your system for long. I personally take one capsule two to three times per day.

Alpha Lipoic Acid

Alpha lipoic acid is a super supplement with multiple benefits. It is well known for being a natural treatment for diabetes and peripheral neuropathy. It helps to support nerve function and reduce nerve pain. It has been shown to lower triglycerides and help with insulin resistance and weight loss.[172] It is called the "universal antioxidant" because it is both water and fat soluble, so it is well-absorbed by your body either with food or on an empty stomach. Alpha lipoic acid helps boost your production of glutathione, neutralize free radicals, and slow the aging process.

It also helps prevent memory loss and cognitive decline. Many medical professionals recommend it to patients suffering neuron damage, motor impairment, and memory loss. It is **one of only a few antioxidants that can cross the blood brain barrier**, and this results in unique benefits for brain health. It can protect delicate brain and nerve tissue. It can also help prevent strokes and various brain problems including dementia in older adults. Eye benefits are another major plus for those taking alpha lipoic acid. It is often recommended to slow the progression of retinal damage, macular degeneration, cataracts, glaucoma and more.

Recommendations

You can get alpha lipoic acid from certain foods, but supplements are needed for a therapeutic dose, especially for those with diabetes, insulin resistance, vision, or neurological disorders. A typical dose is 300–600 mg daily.

Antioxidants – Beta-carotene (Vitamin A Precursor), Vitamin C, Vitamin E, and Selenium

People with hypothyroidism commonly have a higher level of free radical production and lower antioxidant levels. High cholesterol levels, high blood sugar, and metabolic syndrome are also more common in people with hypothyroidism, and all these conditions can increase oxidative stress.

Oxidative stress in the body can contribute to many illnesses, including Hashimoto's, rheumatoid arthritis, chronic inflammation, cardiovascular disease, cataracts, and other vision problems. Antioxidants are essential for healthy vision. Antioxidants neutralize free radicals in your body, which protects you from damage caused by oxidation which can damage our cells.

Recommendations

Remember that you can look up the ORAC values of foods, which is a score of antioxidant content. Some of the foods with the highest antioxidant values include chaga mushroom, cacao, vanilla bean, cinnamon, turmeric, peppermint leaves, rosemary spice, oregano, basil, curry, and cumin. So, spice up your cooking with these mighty herbs.

The most commonly known antioxidant supplements include vitamin A, vitamin C, vitamin E, and selenium. Keep in mind that the dosage is key. The RDA for vitamin C is only 60 mg, but it becomes an antioxidant at doses above 600 mg. You must take doses of 600 mg and up to get the antioxidant benefits. The RDA for vitamin E is only 10 mg, but it becomes an antioxidant at a dose of 200–400 mg. The RDA for selenium is 70 mcg, but it should be taken at a dose of 200–400 mcg for people with Hashimoto's.

For vitamin A, I recommend being tested before taking any supplements with vitamin A or beta carotene. You must be careful, because having too much vitamin A in your body over a long period of time can cause serious illness. I do not supplement with beta carotene or vitamin A because my blood work showed a high result. If you are low in vitamin A, I recommend taking a natural form of mixed carotenes if you are not getting enough through your diet.

Glutathione and NAC

Glutathione is known as the body's master antioxidant. While other antioxidants such as vitamin E and vitamin C come from the food you eat, glutathione is produced by the cells in your body, especially the liver. Less glutathione is produced as you get older starting at around 45 to 50 years old. Glutathione is a tripeptide (a peptide made from three amino acids). N-Acetyl Cysteine (NAC), L-Glutamine, and Glycine are all natural precursors to glutathione.

Glutathione helps protect you from many health problems. It is critical in almost every system of the body. Glutathione provides these benefits:

- Detoxifies the liver
- Neutralizes toxins in the body
- Transports mercury out of the brain
- Eliminates free radicals
- Repairs and supports production of DNA
- Reduces inflammation and oxidative stress
- Supports the entire immune system and increases white blood cells
- Prevents or lessens the effects of these conditions: Dementia, Alzheimer's disease, chronic fatigue, liver disease, cancer, arthritis, heart disease, and respiratory illness

Glutathione Lowers Homocysteine

Glutathione can lower homocysteine levels. **Elevated homocysteine** is a risk factor for cardiovascular disease, stroke, cognitive decline, dementia, and Alzheimer's disease in older adults.[173] Elevated homocysteine levels affect people more as they get older.

N-Acetyl Cysteine (NAC) helps to replenish glutathione levels in your cells. Taking oral NAC supplements reduced homocysteine levels in people in several clinical trials. The dose of NAC given in these trials varied from 600 mg to 4,000 mg per day. All dosages led to a significant decline in homocysteine levels. The more NAC people took, the more their homocysteine level went down. Some people experienced a 50 percent reduction in their homocysteine levels.[174]

NAC Lowers Toxicity

Many people with Hashimoto's have an impaired ability to eliminate toxins. This makes it more likely for them to have an accumulation of toxins. Toxicity is a major root cause of this illness. You can eat foods that help your body make glutathione, but when dealing with toxicity, you must provide your body with extra help to make glutathione. Increasing your glutathione levels is an important part of helping your body eliminate toxins.

NAC vs. Glutathione

What should you take? Liposomal glutathione or NAC? There have been issues with glutathione supplements not being as bioavailable as NAC. Glutathione supplements have been known to break down in the digestive tract. The liposomal form of glutathione is considered more bioavailable. You can take NAC instead, which is absorbed in the gastrointestinal tract, goes to the liver, and gets converted to cysteine, which the liver uses to produce glutathione. However, companies make better products all the time. I recently found a formula with liposomal glutathione, phosphatidylcholine, L-cysteine, L-Glutamic acid, L-Glycine, milk thistle, vitamin C, alpha lipoic acid, and trimethylglycine. That's a winning combination! Apply the following recommendations when taking the product of your choice.

Recommendations

- Take NAC daily 30 minutes before or two hours after meals. It can be taken:
  - **Orally** (capsules)—The daily recommended dose is 600–1,800 mg of NAC
  - **Intravenously**—NAC IV infusion therapy is offered at medical spas. The cost averages at about $100 per infusion. NAC is given by IV for brain health, fertility, and respiratory health (such as asthma, cystic fibrosis, pulmonary fibrosis, COPD, or chronic

bronchitis). IV NAC is also given for weight loss. It has the potential to balance blood sugar levels, reduce inflammation, and improve insulin resistance.

- Meditate regularly. People that practice meditation have 20 percent higher glutathione levels.[175]
- Get enough rest. Adequate sleep can help increase glutathione levels.
- Eat foods that are rich in glutathione, such as asparagus, avocado, beef, broccoli, garlic, chicken, brussels sprouts, and cauliflower.
- Eat foods high in sulfur (such as garlic, onions, legumes, and nuts). They are known to boost your natural production of glutathione.

Carbon (C60)

Carbon 60 (C60) is a supplement that is not widely known, but it is gaining notoriety in the supplement world. Its benefits include everything from increasing your lifespan to preventing arthritis pain and reducing overall inflammation.

C60 has special dome-shaped carbon atoms with sixty electrons on each one that are donated to neutralize free radicals. This makes it a powerful antioxidant. C60 has a strong ability to cause apoptosis, which is the natural cell death of cancer cells. In addition, it supports the liver, kidneys, intestines, and your body as a whole.

What is carbon C60? The C60 molecule was discovered in 1985. It is made up of 60 carbon molecules, which is how it gets its name. These carbon molecules form 12 pentagons (a shape with five equal sides) and 20 hexagons (a shape with six equal sides). This combination of pentagons and hexagons turns C60 into the shape of a soccer ball. The official name of C60 is buckminsterfullerene, but they are commonly referred to as buckyballs because of their round shape.

C60 was initially studied for the unique properties described above but later was studied for its health benefits and industrial applications. The researchers who discovered it were awarded a Nobel Prize in 1996. In 2011, a team led by researcher Fathi Moussa researched C60 to test for potential toxicity. What they discovered was that C60 is one of the **least toxic** substances known to man. Not only does it appear to be non-toxic, it's also been shown to be **anti-toxic**.

Moussa ran a study with three groups of rats. One group was given C60 with olive oil. The second group was given plain water. The third group was given plain olive oil. See the results below.

Group	Given Daily	Result at End of Study
1	**C60** Olive Oil	**100 percent** of the **C60** olive oil-fed rats were still alive! They continued to live on beyond their lifespans. In fact, the natural lifespans of the group one C60-fed rats increased by as much as **95 percent**. They lived almost twice as long as they normally would.
2	Plain water	All the water-fed rats were dead.
3	Plain olive oil	67 percent of the group 3 plain olive oil group were dead.

The C60 olive oil-fed rats **lived almost twice** as long as their normal lifespan! These are incredibly exciting results indeed with potential for extending longevity!

Of course, this finding does not automatically map to humans. There's a lot more to growing old than just free radical damage. Everyone is predisposed to different ailments and conditions, so there's no guarantee of anything. More human studies are needed. However, there is plenty of research that suggests taking a C60 supplement can provide numerous health benefits, including:

- Reduced obesity and metabolic syndrome symptoms (heart disease, stroke, diabetes)
- Reduced inflammation, particularly in arthritis patients[176]
- Prevention of osteoarthritis[177]
- Protection against UV damage to skin[178]

Recommendations

C60 products are in a base of olive oil. I personally take the Wolfe-Carbon-Detox liquid C60 product. Take as directed on the label.

Black Seed Oil (Nigella Sativa)

Nigella sativa, also known as black cumin seed, has been used for thousands of years to treat many ailments. Nigella sativa is described in ancient medical and religious literature, and even the Bible. When its seeds are cold-pressed, a golden oil is extracted.

There are more than 1900 scientific publications on nigella sativa. A review of this research found that nigella sativa can be used to improve the following conditions, many of which are common in people with Hashimoto's:

- Metabolic syndrome—Helps to achieve and maintain a healthy weight
- Type 2 diabetes—Decreases both fasting and post-meal blood sugar, and long-term glucose (HbA1c) levels.
- High cholesterol—Decreases blood lipid levels
- Rheumatoid arthritis—Decreases swollen joints and morning stiffness
- Viral infections
- High blood pressure
- Nonalcoholic fatty liver disease (NAFLD)
- Chronic inflammation
- Cardiovascular and kidney health
- Reduced level of arsenic by 70 percent

- Helps treat polycystic ovary syndrome (PCOS) and menopausal symptoms
- Treats skin, gut, wound, MRSA, respiratory, hepatitis, and candida infections
- Dissolves kidney stones
- Helps treat dermatitis, psoriasis, eczema, acne, and vitiligo
- Helps improve asthma, allergies, and lung function[179]

Thyroid Benefits

Studies suggest that **nigella sativa helps reverse Hashimoto's disease** and promotes the health of the thyroid. In a study of 40 patients with Hashimoto's disease, TSH, thyroid antibodies, and vascular endothelial growth factor decreased and the thyroid hormone T3 level increased. In addition, patients experienced significantly **reduced body weight** and body mass index (BMI). Researchers suggest it may be an effective treatment for autoimmune diseases in general.[180]

Recommendations

Select a brand with a golden color and strong scent to ensure you are buying a quality product. Take the recommended dose (per your practitioner) in soft gel form, not liquid. The taste is horrible. Although I was very impressed and hopeful after reading the research, my personal experience with black seed oil was not good. The first product I tried was in liquid form, and it was like drinking motor oil. I continued to taste it for hours afterwards. That bottle ended up in the garbage. I just recently tried it again after reviewing the research. I took two soft gels after eating. I had some mild burping, bringing up the strong taste of the oil. I tried again after a meal and I not only had the mild burping with the reminder of the taste, I also had discomfort near my sternum. I'm sharing this experience to warn my readers. Maybe it would better to take it in the middle of your meal and take only one soft gel at a time. The product I tried is highly rated. Perhaps I am very sensitive, but I think it is important to warn my readers that this product is very strong.

Probiotics

It is important to keep your microbiome replenished with beneficial bacteria because it is an important part of your intestinal barrier and your immune system. Probiotics help prevent the growth of harmful bacteria by competing for nutrients. They help your digestion and the absorption of nutrients, and they help reverse leaky gut. As mentioned in Chapter 10, the probiotic Lactobacillus rhamnosus GG was shown to strengthen the intestinal barrier.

Certain probiotics, including Lactobacillus plantarum have been found to reduce absorption of heavy metals and in turn reduce inflammation and intestinal permeability.[181]

Eating fermented foods is a great way to consume probiotics but if you don't eat them often, taking quality probiotic supplements daily provides you with a more reliable source of probiotics.

Recommendations

If you've never taken probiotics, you may want to start with a 10 billion CFU probiotic and progress to a higher dose over time. High dose (50 billion CFU), multi-strain probiotics can be very helpful for people with Hashimoto's.

General Recommendations for Supplementation

It can be confusing to choose among the plethora of vitamins, herbs, minerals, supplements, shakes, juices, and nutraceuticals on the market. I've studied these types of products and used many of them for decades, beginning in the 1990s when my mother was struggling with various health issues.

There are many excellent nutritional drinks, foods, and thyroid formulas to choose from. Read labels and avoid any allergens or artificial sweeteners. I do not recommend taking tablets because they are harder for the body to break down and sometimes do not fully dissolve and get assimilated by the body.

Premium brands are known for their quality and are usually more costly. While premium products often have superior and more trustworthy ingredient sources, I don't believe in spending more than necessary. Some people think that it must be costly to work well, but that's not always the case. As an example, I have used a brand of Alpha lipoic acid (ALA) that costs $20 for 120 servings. I worked well for me because I used to get cramps and spasms in my feet, and it eliminated that problem. If I didn't take it, the cramps would return. As an opposite example, I paid $100 for a four-ounce bottle of CBD oil. It was a highly rated brand. I took it daily until it was gone, hoping it would help reduce my inflammation and pain in my neck and shoulders. It did nothing. I am currently trying a new brand of ALA (also $20) that boasts high bioavailability. It includes two top grade forms of ALA including the more absorbable form of ALA (S-ALA and R-ALA), as well as vitamin B1 and benfotiamine. This demonstrates that you can always level up with better products even if what you have is working.

Should you take a multivitamin? I generally avoid them unless they are designed or recommended for people with Hashimoto's or MTHFR gene mutations. It must be gluten free. It should have methylated B vitamins, probiotics, and immune-modulating herbs. It should be rich in minerals with a good amount of selenium, zinc, copper, potassium, magnesium, chromium, and molybdenum. Some supplements should be taken separately to ensure you get a large enough dose, especially when it comes to the nutrients that people with Hashimoto's are commonly deficient in. I do take nutritional products with multiple ingredients focused on a certain goal and I always carefully review the ingredients and make sure quality versions of nutrients are included. For example, B12 and folate must be the methylated form. I also pay attention to fillers and capsule type, and I always ensure they are non-GMO and do not contain soy, gluten, and other allergens.

Do you have to take every supplement every single day? No. Do you have to stick to the same supplements forever? No. I think it is good to change your routine through the stages of your life and to address specific health challenges. Certain supplements are important to take regularly, such as vitamin C, vitamin D, selenium, and magnesium. Others are meant to address certain health conditions and may only need to be taken for a short time. For example, you may take a course of parasite-killing supplements for a few weeks or months, or you might take a course of antiviral supplements for a few weeks.

The good thing about taking supplements is that it makes you drink plenty of water. I suggest keeping supplements that you take with food separate from those you take on an empty stomach. Sometimes, it's hard to take them all each day. I find it easier to take them with a warm herbal tea. There are several brands that I recommend to clients and feature in blog articles. If you don't have time to research on your own, consult with a health professional that is well-versed and experienced with a variety of nutritional products and medical conditions.

CHAPTER 14

Tumor Shrinkers and Detoxifiers

"Calcification is the hardening of body tissues by calcium salts or deposits. Although calcification itself is not considered a disease, it has been shown to be a significant contributing factor in nearly every known illness and aging condition, including heart disease, kidney stones, gallstones, chronic inflammation, arthritis, cancers, cataracts, eczema, psoriasis, and even wrinkles."
– David Wolfe

This chapter describes several clinically proven natural cancer treatments that detoxify the body, prevent calcification, and shrink cysts and tumors. I used all but two of the items described in this chapter. I used several of them to shrink my thyroid nodules and detoxify heavy metals and other toxins.

Cancer is a concern for everyone and certainly becomes a more urgent concern if you are diagnosed with thyroid nodules.

We are all exposed to pesticides, environmental pollutants, heavy metals, air pollution, and many toxic ingredients in the foods we eat and products we use. There is no avoiding it, so detoxing is a smart and effective way to protect your health and prevent cysts, nodules, and tumors. Sadly, the poisoning starts in infancy.

Toxins in Newborns

One of the most tragic aspects of this problem is that our unborn children already bear a toxic burden. A 2004 study by the Environmental Working Group identified 287 industrial chemicals in babies' umbilical-cord blood. Of these, 180 are known to cause cancer and 217 are toxic to the brain and nervous system!

It does not occur to parents of brand-new beautiful babies that they need to be detoxed to prevent disease but it's a good idea to do so and there are safe ways to do it. One of them is a simple clay bath. Babies and children are at risk. We all are. That is a sad but true fact. There are several ways to reduce that risk. Reducing the chemical load in children will help them to learn better. It will help their brains to function better and that is turn will likely help their behavior. Imagine thinking you had a bad child due to poor behavior and then you find out through testing that your child is toxic with mercury poisoning. Please help your child detox and support their detoxification by providing clean and healthy nutritious food. They deserve a cleaner world!

In recent laboratory tests, glyphosate, the main ingredient in Bayer-Monsanto's Roundup, was detected in **all** 21 oat-based cereal and snack products tested. This includes several varieties of Cheerios and Nature Valley products. All these products contained unsafe levels of glyphosate for children. You can read the full report to find out what foods to avoid.[182]

Although concerns about Roundup date back to the 1980s, nothing was done until 2021. Courts are now listening, and judgements totaling over $10 million have been ordered, many for victims of Hodgkin's Lymphoma. Victims are coming forward and winning awards.[183] Bayer plans to remove glyphosate from *residential* Roundup beginning in 2023. I never thought I would see the day! Hopefully, they won't create another dangerous pesticide or herbicide that takes decades to take off the market.

In this chapter, you will learn about safe treatments and natural substances that can be used to detoxify everyone, including children and adults.

Modified Citrus Pectin (MCP)

Modified citrus pectin (MCP) is the primary and possibly the most beneficial part of my thyroid-nodule-shrinking regime. I used the Pectasol-C brand, made by EcoNugenics. I took six capsules three times a day. I also used the powder version. Buying the powder is less expensive than buying capsules so now I choose to mix the Pectasol-C powder into a cup of organic applesauce. I continue to take MCP for the incredible array of benefits it offers.

The proven benefits of MCP are outlined in this chapter. MCP is recognized as one of the most advanced, broad-spectrum nutraceuticals of our time. It could potentially save or prolong your life or that of your loved ones.

What is MCP?

Modified citrus pectin (MCP) is made from pectin, which is found in the white pith of citrus peels of fruits such as lemons, limes, and oranges. It is called "modified citrus pectin" because the pectin is altered using a special enzyme and PH-controlled process to make it a lower molecular weight so that the body can absorb it more easily in the gut and the bloodstream. The original form of MCP that Dr. Issac Eliaz helped develop over 25 years ago contains the correct size and structure that is clinically proven in many studies to be effective.

You may be familiar with *apple* pectin. It is often used by people as a supplement to increase fiber intake and support intestinal health. Apple pectin is a type of soluble fiber that may potentially improve cholesterol, blood pressure, gut health, and bowel stability. Apple pectin has a larger molecular weight than MCP. It is used as a source of fiber and mainly stays in the intestinal track and helps push food through the digestive system. MCP in contrast, with its lower molecular weight, enters the blood circulation from the digestive tract and binds to toxins and other types of cells to reduce their harmful effects.

MCP is now referred to by physicians as the **best-kept secret in integrative medicine**. It is getting a lot of recognition and respect. MCP has been shown to prevent and improve cancer, remove heavy metals, treat fatty liver, and prevent fibrosis and cardiovascular disease (including arteriosclerosis). There are over 80 published studies that demonstrate the capability of MCP to block the harmful effects of excess galectin-3 cells.

The Survival Protein: Galectin-3

Galectins are carbohydrate-binding proteins that are involved in many of your bodily functions, including inflammation and immune response. There are different types of galectins, but the most studied is galectin-3. Galectin-3 cells can become elevated due to illness, injury, or regular aging. When they grow out of control, they become a key factor in the development of degenerative diseases such as cancer, heart disease, obesity, depression, and more.

What is Galectin-3?

Galectin-3 is a carbohydrate-binding protein in the body that plays roles in immunity, cell development, and repair. Galectin-3 is beneficial inside the cell, and in small amounts outside the cell. However, it can have devastating effects if it multiplies out of control. This can happen due to illness, injury, or just regular aging. Excess galectin-3 fuels chronic inflammation and causes widespread harmful effects in the body. In the case of cancer, galectin-3 cells multiply out of control and form tumors. That's where MCP comes in. It prevents those cells from multiplying and clumping together to form tumors.

Galectin-3 protein is the focus of one of the fastest growing fields in medical research today. It is referred to as the "Survival Protein" by Dr. Isaac Eliaz, MD in his book, *The Survival Paradox: Reversing the Hidden Cause of Aging and Chronic Disease*. Over 3,000 published studies show that today's most life-threatening and inflammatory conditions are driven by one common culprit: Galectin-3 protein.

When we are sick, injured, or experiencing stressors, galectin-3 cells are generated and kick into action repairing the injuries as part of our body's innate survival response. However, if the galectin-3 activity continues after the threat is gone, these galectin-3 cells can multiply out of control and cause inflammation and **fibrosis** instead of healing. Fibrosis leads to scar tissue build-up and hardening of blood vessels, tissues, and organ systems. This can affect the brain, joints, and the cardiovascular system.

What is Fibrosis?

When you have an injury or a disease that causes damage to the body (such as arterial linings, kidneys, or liver), connective tissue is created and adheres to the area of damage to repair it. Simply put, it is an exaggerated wound healing response that can interfere with the normal functioning of the diseased organ or tissue. It's also known as calcification.

Thousands of published studies show that when galectin-3 multiplies out of control, it can lead to degenerative conditions.

Conditions Correlated with Excess Galectin-3	
Inflammation and tissue fibrosis (uncontrolled scar tissue build up)	Immune suppression
Cancer growth and metastasis	Arthritis
Cardiovascular disease and arteriosclerosis	Metabolic syndrome
Kidney disease	Obesity
Premature aging	Neurological degeneration
Depression	Organ dysfunction

Only one medicine has a proven ability to stop and reverse the harmful effects of galectin-3. It is a natural medicine. It is **modified citrus pectin**, and specifically the Pectasol-C product from the EcoNugenics company. Pectasol-C is the brand that has been used in clinical studies. It is created with an advanced enzymatic process that breaks the long chain molecules of regular citrus pectin to produce a much smaller size and structure of citrus pectin. With this smaller molecular structure, the MCP is able to enter your circulation and bind to rogue galectin-3, safely disarming it. Although other unstudied brands of modified citrus pectin are available, I prefer, trust, and recommend the only researched form of MCP, Pectasol-C.

MCP Benefits

A significant number of published studies show that MCP inhibits galectin-3. It has been proven to bind to galectin-3, block cancer cells from clumping together to form tumors, prevent angiogenesis, and reduce metastasis. This is a massive scientific development. And to bolster that finding even more, it is completely non-toxic and has a multitude of other significant health benefits.

Cancer

In relation to cancer, having excess galectin-3 contributes to:

- Growth of new tumors
- Metastasis—spread of cancer to other organs or tissues[184]
- Angiogenesis—growth of blood vessels that supply tumors[185]
- Poor outcomes for cancer patients

Galectin-3 has been studied as a potential therapeutic target in several cancers, such as breast cancer, prostate cancer, colon cancer, gastric cancer, and multiple myeloma.[186] MCP inhibits galectin-3 and is known for its potential to prevent and treat many types of cancer, including the reversal of breast cancer.[187] MCP reduced tumor growth, angiogenesis, and metastasis in mice treated with MCP.[188] PectaSol-C was also shown to block the spread of prostate cancer and lower PSA scores by inhibiting galectin-3.[189]

MCP has been shown to effectively target multiple processes that lead to cancer metastasis, including the promotion of apoptosis (death of cancer cells). MCP also enhances apoptosis induced by cytotoxic drugs, which means that it can potentially increase the effectiveness of conventional chemotherapy.[190] MCP is also **safe for dogs**. It has a very low risk of bad reactions because it's basically food.[191] Tumor growth and metastasis was reduced in human and canine tumors by using MCP.[192]

Heavy Metals Detoxification

MCP helps with detoxification by removing heavy metals, environmental toxins, and radioactive isotopes from the body. Three clinical studies have shown MCP can be used as a safe binder and chelator of heavy metals. **MCP reduces blood levels of lead, mercury, arsenic, cadmium, and others**. A review of five case studies showed that toxic heavy metals were reduced by 74% average without side effects in people using PectaSol (MCP) alone or combined with alginates (polysaccharides found in brown algae).[193]

MCP is also a safe treatment for children who have been exposed to lead. Treatment with MCP for children hospitalized with lead toxicity resulted in dramatically decreased levels of lead in the children's blood, and increased levels of lead excreted in the children's urine.[194]

An important concern about some chelation substances is that they may remove beneficial minerals from the body. However, MCP studies have shown that when using MCP, the **minerals are preserved in the body**.[247]

Treatment for Cardiovascular Disease

Galectin-3 is now used as a biomarker for heart failure because excess galectin-3 cells cause inflammatory conditions and fibrosis in the cardiovascular system. An increasing number of research studies are looking at the ability of MCP to reverse cardiovascular disease by blocking galectin-3.[246]

Treatment for Fatty Liver

MCP helps liver health in several ways. In a 2021 study, MCP reduced fat accumulation in Non-Alcoholic Fatty Liver (NAFL) disease.[195] Another study published in 2022 showed promise for liver cancer. Treatment with MCP induced cell death (apoptosis) of liver cancer (HepG2) cells.[196]

Treatment for Inflammatory Diseases

The Pectasol-C form of MCP is recognized in the scientific community as one of the most advanced, broad-spectrum nutraceuticals, with over seventy clinical studies demonstrating its effectiveness.

Multiple studies have shown that MCP helps to treat the following conditions that involve inflammation and fibrosis.

Conditions Helped by Modified Citrus Pectin			
Cardiovascular disease	Kidney disease	Diabetes	Sepsis
Liver cirrhosis	Insulin resistance	Arthritis	Cancer

Recommendations

In *The Survival Paradox*, Dr. Isaac Eliaz, MD., provides recommended nutritional protocols for major conditions, including autoimmune support, liver disease, cardiovascular and kidney support, arthritis, and Lyme disease. For each condition he provides a protocol with various supplements and the recommended dosage of MCP powder, which is usually 7.5 grams, twice a day (dose may be adjusted for weight). MCP can also be taken in the form of capsules or chewable tablets. Dr. Eliaz also recommends intermittent fasting and a low-glycemic anti-inflammatory diet.

If you have thyroid nodules, I suggest taking a 5-gram dose three times a day, or a 7.5-gram dose twice a day.

Zeolite (Clinoptilolite) Powder

Zeolite is a silica-based volcanic ash (mineral) that forms over time when ash and lava from volcanoes chemically react with sea water. Zeolite is a collective name for several minerals and chemical compounds within the group known as silicates. Zeolite is a binder and a natural "adsorbant." Adsorption means that molecules stick to the surface of an object as opposed to dissolving into it (absorption).

The zeolite mineral is negatively charged by nature. Toxins, such as heavy metals, radioactive elements, BPA, mycotoxins (mold), glyphosate, pollutants, and pesticides, have a positive charge. Zeolite is attracted to the toxins like a magnet and pulls them into its structure. Harmful toxins become trapped in zeolite's cage-like structure and are then safely and gently carried out of the body. This is an advantage over many detoxification products because it prevents the toxins from recirculating throughout the body and causing detoxification die-off effects. One of the best aspects of zeolite is that it does not remove your minerals and positive elements because they do not have a positive charge and thus do not get attracted into the zeolite cages.

There are several types of zeolites. There are industrial forms of zeolite used for environmental cleanup purposes and agricultural forms used for soil management. The clinoptilolite form of zeolite is the type used internally by people to safely detoxify harmful heavy metals. Clinoptilolite has been widely studied in veterinary and human medicine. It resembles a silky clay powder and blends easily with water or any beverage.[197] It helps support the body's natural ability to detoxify without the harsh, unwanted side effects often associated with detox.

Benefits of Zeolite (Clinoptilolite)

The benefits of zeolite (clinoptilolite) powder are as follows.

Chelates Heavy Metals

Zeolite can help reduce and chelate several heavy metals and other chemicals that accumulate in your body.

Heavy Metals and Chemicals Reduced by Zeolite		
Arsenic	Cadmium	Cesium
Chromium	Copper	Cobalt
Lead	Manganese	Mercury
Molybdenum	Nickel	Uranium
PCBs	Pesticides	Herbicides

Studies have confirmed that zeolite clinoptilolite binds to and removes heavy metals such as lead, arsenic, and mercury.[198][199][200]

Antimicrobial Effects

Zeolite clinoptilolite has antibacterial properties against many common infections, including the following.

Infections Improved by Zeolite Powder		
Escherichia coli (E Coli)	Clostridium difficile	Salmonella pullorum
Staphylococcus aureus (Staph)	Streptococcus gordonii (Strep)	Methicillin-Resistant Staphylococcus Aureus (MRSA)
Porphyromonas gingivalis (main cause of periodontitis)		

Antifungal Effects

Zeolite has antifungal properties against candida albicans.

Antiviral Effects

Zeolite has antiviral effects due to its ability to adsorb viral cells into its cage-like structure. Zeolite also appears to block the replication of viruses.

Anecdotal case studies have reported people using zeolite powder have been healed from herpes zoster, rheumatoid arthritis, multiple sclerosis, hepatitis C, and the common cold and flu.

Gastrointestinal Disease

Zeolite helps to alleviate gastritis and diarrhea. Zeolite also improves liver function, indirectly improving elimination of pesticides, herbicides, and xenoestrogens.

Periodontal Disease

Zeolite nanoparticles can help prevent periodontal diseases, such as gingivitis by reducing growth of harmful bacteria and plaque. Additionally, zeolite can lessen bad breath by reducing bacteria.

Improves Cholesterol and Blood Lipid Levels

In a clinical trial of 41 patients, micronized zeolite lowered blood levels of the "bad" cholesterol (LDL) and blood lipids and raised the "good" cholesterol (HDL). After eight weeks of taking a dose of 6–9 g daily, their cholesterol values improved by 20–25 percent.[201]

Recommendations

Zeolite Pure zeolite powder and Heiltropfen zeolite powder are brands that I use. Zeolite Pure is micronized from 0-40 μm, with most of the small particle size under 7 μm. The small particle size allows for a deep cellular cleanse, while the larger sizes help provide cleansing effects throughout the body and in the GI tract and colon. The Heiltropfen brand from Norway is ultrafine with <20 μm.

There are liquid zeolite products, but I choose not to use them because I think the liquid products are too diluted and contain too small of a dose. In fact, recent studies have shown the powder form is more effective.[202] I have used the powder form on several occasions. The first time, I put a tablespoon in my smoothie each day for two weeks. It made a big difference in how I felt. After two weeks of use, I felt a heightened sense of clarity, well-being, and happiness. Note that prior to beginning zeolite, I had taken MCP for several weeks, so perhaps the two combined treatments resulted in the significant effect I experienced.

Importance of Dosing: The traditional method of starting with a low dose and gradually increasing does not apply with zeolite and can actually cause a serious reaction. You need a large enough amount to bind to the toxins and not allow them to redistribute throughout the body. When taking zeolite, it grabs onto toxic (positively charged) elements, and those toxins get stirred up and start releasing into the circulation. Having a large enough dose of zeolite ensures that the extra zeolite "cages" grab (or encapsulate) whatever gets stirred into circulation.

The lower the dose, the higher the, the higher the chance of a detox reaction. In fact, people that experience a detox reaction from taking zeolite are advised to take a higher dose immediately, and after doing so, reported their detox symptoms lifting within minutes. Some sources recommend a once daily dose of 15 grams (two tablespoons). The more toxic you are, the higher the dose you need.

Note: Zeolite should not be taken together with prescription medications or other supplements because it can potentially bind to them and reduce their effect. Also, remember while taking zeolite powder to drink more water than usual and eat plenty of vegetables to keep your bowels moving. It's okay to take if you have consumed alcohol. In fact, it absorbs alcohol and is used to prevent and treat hangovers.[203]

Activated Charcoal

Activated charcoal is a multipurpose remedy. It is a binder that is best when created from coconut shells or peat (vegetable matter) and ground into ultra-fine powder. This is NOT the charcoal that you use in the barbeque.

Activated charcoal has a negative electric charge and it attracts and removes positively charged compounds. These compounds include molds, mycotoxins, bacteria, heavy metals, and toxic metabolic byproducts of unwanted microbes and other organisms. This is helpful for people exposed to mold, dental amalgams, and other toxins. Activated charcoal is used for the safe and effective treatment of poisoning and drug overdoses. In fact, emergency trauma centers use it all over the world.

Activated charcoal is also an excellent solution if you overindulge in food or drink. Whether you've eaten too much greasy food, been exposed to harmful bacteria, or drank too much alcohol, activated charcoal can help "mop up" the toxic aftermath and help you feel better faster. It also helps with diarrhea, gas, and bloating.

If taking a charcoal supplement, it is best to take it on an empty stomach when using it to detox. Drink plenty of water and make sure your bowels are moving. Remember, activated charcoal is a binder. In addition to binding to toxins, it can also bind with other supplements or medications and reduce their effectiveness, so it's best taken alone. Do not take it within an hour of prescription medications or supplements.

A new ozonated form of activated charcoal has become available. According to Dr. Edward Group of Global Healing, ozonation can make activated charcoal up to 10X more effective when it comes to improving your health. When activated charcoal combines with ozone, it enhances the charcoal's already impressive adsorptive properties, enhancing its potential detoxification benefits. In fact, Dr. Group says that ozonated charcoal is the only thing that can remove microplastics from the body.

The ozonation process helps to provide additional benefits that make ozonated activated charcoal far more capable of trapping toxins and impurities, and supporting overall health. I anticipate research on ozonated charcoal is forthcoming, but at this point, there seems to be far more clinical evidence for the benefits of modified citrus pectin and zeolite (Clinoptilolite).

Gerson Therapy

Dr. Max Gerson developed the Gerson Therapy in the 1920s and it is still being used today to save lives. It is a natural treatment protocol that activates the body's innate ability to heal itself by treating the underlying cause of degenerative disease, which is often toxicity and nutritional deficiency. The Gerson protocol consists of an organic, plant-based diet, raw juices, colon therapy, and natural supplements. The Gerson Institute is located in San Diego, CA. You can learn more on the Gerson Institute website.[204]

Sulforaphane

Sulforaphane is a sulfur-rich compound found in cruciferous vegetables like broccoli, cabbage, cauliflower, bok choy, and kale. Steaming these vegetables for one to three minutes is the best way to optimize sulforaphane levels.

One of the richest sources of sulforaphane is found in broccoli sprouts, which are three-to-five-day-old broccoli plants. They are also a rich source of fiber, protein, vitamins, and minerals, but the most impressive benefits are due to sulforaphane. Studies show that sulforaphane has 82 percent bioavailability, which means a high amount of it is easily absorbed.

Sulforaphane can also reduce viral load. The number of viruses in a person's blood is called the "viral load." After recovering from viruses, our blood still contains viral cells. Keeping your viral load low is a great way to help your immune system.

Autoimmune Disease and Inflammation

Sulforaphane has another benefit that is especially helpful for those with autoimmune disease. People with autoimmune disease often have chronic or systemic inflammation. Sulforaphane works against inflammation by activating the "Nrf2" pathway, which combats oxidative stress and inflammation throughout the entire body. Consuming sulforaphane activates Nrf2, which helps decrease systemic inflammation throughout your whole body.

Cancer

Sulforaphane was shown in several studies to act against pancreatic, prostate, breast, lung, cervical, and colorectal cancers.[205]

Slows Aging

Sulforaphane helps to slow down aging. As we age, our metabolic processes slow down, we lose collagen, we can't repair wounds and build muscle as well, and we build up oxidative damage. Nrf2 production slows down which allows more free radicals to build up. You can increase your Nrf2 production to break down those free radicals with sulforaphane.

Diabetes

Sulforaphane also helps with diabetes. In a study of people with diabetes, sulforaphane was taken in the form of concentrated broccoli sprout extract. Subjects that took sulforaphane reduced their fasting blood sugar levels by 6.5 percent and had improved hemoglobin A1C.[206]

Recommendations

Sometimes, I grow broccoli sprouts in my kitchen and I either put them in a smoothie or eat them with chopped romaine and raspberry vinaigrette. However, it's not a food I enjoy eating daily, so sometimes I take a concentrated dose via capsules. You can purchase capsules with concentrated broccoli sprout powder.

Chamomile Tea to Prevent Thyroid Cancer and other Tumors

Chamomile is an excellent medicinal tea for anyone with thyroid disease. It is rich in apigenin, which is especially beneficial for Hashimoto's and other autoimmune diseases. Apigenin is a type of flavonoid or phytochemical that exists in many types of plants including chamomile, parsley, onions, rosemary, and many other fruits, vegetables, and herbs.

Apigenin is an antioxidant you want to ensure you have in your diet because it has significant anti-inflammatory effects. In fact, consuming antioxidants is one of the best things you can do to lower chronic inflammation. Apigenin has also been shown to modulate your immune system, reduce insulin sensitivity, reduce inflammation, and protect against viruses and cancer.[207]

Apigenin is also an immune modulator! Keeping the immune system in balance is the goal. Apigenin fights oxidative stress, which is a causative factor in the development of cancer. Research has shown that apigenin may inhibit cell growth in many types of tumors (skin, liver, breast, lung, etc.). In addition, apigenin appears to decipher cancerous cells as different from normal cells.

Scientific Proof of Chamomile's Anticancer Benefits

There have been many highly publicized studies on the benefits of black tea and green tea. Green tea is rich in antioxidants and anticancer agents such as catechins. However, each cup contains about 70 mg of caffeine which can stimulate you and interfere with sleep, especially if consumed later in the day. Many studies have focused on the benefits of black and green tea but there are only a few studies on the effects of herbal teas on thyroid disease.

A study published in the European *Journal of Public Health* in 2015 concluded that drinking chamomile tea regularly over a 30-year period **reduced the risk of thyroid cancer in people by 80 percent** compared to those who did not drink tea.[208] More specifically, they found that drinking two to six cups per week of chamomile tea **reduced the risk of any thyroid disease by 74 percent.** They took multiple factors into consideration including age, gender, and BMI. Adjustment for smoking, alcohol, and coffee consumption did not affect the results. That is considered very significant!

More Benefits of Apigenin

More impressive benefits of apigenin include:

Supports cardiovascular health. Reduces blood pressure and inflammation. Animal studies showed that apigenin has cardioprotective effects in rats with heart damage and can lessen the severity of myocarditis and prevent myocarditis from leading to heart failure.[209]

Fights cancer cells. Apigenin has beneficial effects for virtually all types of cancer because it slows the rate of cancer cell growth and increases the rate of apoptosis (tumor cell death). Apigenin fights cancer at every stage. It has been found to inhibit the initiation, progression, and metastasis of tumors.[210]

Diabetes. Apigenin can increase insulin sensitivity by stimulating the metabolism of glucose and helping transport it into peripheral limbs and tissues throughout the body.

Treats Alzheimer's disease and amnesia. In several studies, apigenin was found to improve memory and overall cognition in patients with Alzheimer's disease and amnesia. In Alzheimer's patients, it was shown to decrease the formation of the beta-amyloid plaque and reduce the amount of fibrillar amyloid deposits.

Reduces inflammation and pain. Apigenin can reduce pain related to inflammatory conditions such as migraine headaches, digestive problems, or infections.

Anti-estrogenic. Apigenin may lower cancer risk for estrogen-related cancers.

Combats depression and anxiety. Apigenin has relaxing and sedative effects. It can also decrease cortisol which helps the body handle stress.

Helps with autoimmunity. Apigenin is a potential therapeutic agent for autoimmune diseases, including multiple sclerosis and lupus. It has anti-inflammatory, anticancer, and antioxidant effects which are helpful to those with autoimmune diseases.

As you can see, there is plentiful evidence of apigenin's benefits, and scientists are calling for studies to examine using apigenin as a therapeutic treatment element for autoimmune disease.

Recommendations

Apigenin can be easily consumed in your daily diet. Although there are supplements with apigenin, it is more stable and bioavailable in plants. So, it's recommended that you get it from foods or spices in your diet and not with supplemental forms. Chamomile tea is an easy way to get apigenin. It is also very relaxing and helpful to ease stress and get to sleep at night. You can also get apigenin by including foods and herbs like parsley, thyme, oregano, cilantro, oranges, red pepper, celery, and onions to your diet. Many fruits and vegetables contain apigenin.

Essiac 4-Herb Tea

Essiac tea is an herbal tea made from four ingredients: burdock root, Indian rhubarb root, sheep sorrel, and slippery elm bark. This is not just any herbal tea. It is herbal medicine. It's a traditional Native American formula that originated with the Ojibwe Indians in Northern Ontario, Canada. A Native American, Ojibwe herbalist approached an English woman and told her he could heal her breast cancer. He gave her the original eight-herb formula and told her how to prepare it. She recovered and shared the recipe.

A cancer nurse named Renee Caisse discovered it in 1922 from a patient who had been treated by the Ojibwe herbalist. After a doctor suggested she test the formula, she treated many patients with multiple ways of administering the herbal formula. She was so successful, the government of Canada and Sloan Kettering got involved. Now named after her, Essiac is Caisse spelled backwards.

The reason there are so many benefits to this herbal medicine is because it helps to clean your liver and kidneys, which are your body's filters. It purifies the blood and removes toxins that can manifest in many different conditions.

Essiac tea became nationwide news in the United States in the 1970s. JFK's doctor treated himself successfully for prostate cancer with Essiac tea and spoke about it on nationwide talk radio. Many testimonials can be found online from people that were helped by using this herbal medicine. There is enormous anecdotal evidence. It was made by the people, for the people. People drink it and they feel better. The only side effect found was vomiting, and it only happened to heavy drinkers. They were detoxing while adding more toxins in. Their body reacted and made them throw up. That's easily avoidable. Don't drink with it.

Some of Essiac's benefits include:

- Purifies the blood
- Removes accumulated toxins in the fat, lymph, bone marrow, bladder, and alimentary canal. This frees up the body for cellular renewal and revitalized health
- Helps the liver with detoxification by converting fatty toxins into water-soluble substances that can be

eliminated through the kidneys
- Neutralizes acids, absorbs toxins in the bowel, and eliminates them
- Reduces, and sometimes eliminates heavy metal deposits in tissues
- Prevents the buildup of excess fatty deposits in artery walls, heart, kidney, and liver
- Improves the functions of the pancreas and spleen by increasing the effectiveness of insulin

It's interesting that some online sources claim that there is a lack of controlled data to prove this herbal medicine's anticancer benefits. This doesn't prove that it doesn't work. It just shows that they haven't conducted controlled studies to prove a specific hypothesis about a specific type of cancer. If you read between the lines, you can deduce that "controlled data" doesn't exist because controlled formal studies are expensive and are not commonly funded and conducted for herbal products and their effects on serious diseases like cancer. Pharmaceutical companies fund the majority of clinical studies with the goal of making profitable medications. There is less funding used to conduct controlled clinical studies to prove specific benefits for herbs, foods, and nutraceuticals.

I saw one study that seemed to discredit Essiac by describing a negative conclusion, but you must read it and decipher for yourself. This study examined the moods in women being treated for breast cancer with traditional chemotherapy.[211] They gave them a very small dose of Essiac, one ounce (30 ml) and then claimed it didn't help their mood. These were young women with aggressive breast cancer. Of course, they would have struggles with their mood. They are facing the fear of death and losing everything. Instead of allowing for mood issues based on a dire diagnosis or toxic treatment, they blame a one ounce a day portion of herbal tea. How convenient and *biased*.

They gave the women **one** ounce. The recommended dose for treating cancer or serious diseases is **two ounces, three times a day**. For less serious conditions, two ounces once a day is recommended. They claimed some women felt worse after taking only one ounce of Essiac tea. How do they know the chemotherapy was not the cause? It is established fact that chemotherapy has *severe* effects on mental and emotional health.[212] Perhaps that is because **chemo medications cross the blood-brain barrier and cause inflammation**. Brain shrinkage (a loss of neurons) has been known to happen as a result of both cancer and chemotherapy.[213] I'm certain that the chemotherapy drugs were the cause of the mood imbalance, not one ounce of herbal tea!

Essiac helps to detox the body and that includes detoxification of medications. In fact, people on chemotherapy can safely take Essiac simultaneously. Many people report that the unpleasant side effects from chemotherapy are reduced when taking Essiac tea.

Anecdotal Evidence

Anecdotal evidence is from personal experience, and it is not always reliable. However, these experiences cannot be disregarded, especially when there are many people experiencing the same thing. There are real stories of people, countless people, over decades, that have recovered from cancer using a variety of safe and natural methods, including Essiac tea. People have had successful results from Essiac for many different conditions.

Empirical Evidence

Empirical evidence is data that is collected from experiments that are run in a controlled environment.

Study Design

When collecting empirical evidence in a clinical trial, the study design should be fair and accurate. Proper dosing is critical. If researchers are biased and administer a smaller dose than indicated for the condition being treated, the results are not going to be valid or accurate. Also, if researchers do not control for variables, such as multiple conditions or medications, the results may not be accurate.

Stanislaw Bryzynski, PHD—Antineoplaston Therapy

One very important and flawed study that comes to mind involved administration of a lower dose than prescribed. It was a study for the safe treatment of deadly brain tumors. Dr. Stanislaw Bryzynski developed a medication in the 1970s after discovering that people with cancer were missing certain peptides that healthy people had in their bodies. He created a safe "antineoplaston" medication to give these peptides to adults and especially children with cancer. He was successfully treating babies and children suffering with malignant brain tumors with antineoplaston therapy. There was finally hope for vulnerable children.

After many efforts to get FDA approval for this medication, the National Institute of Health (NIH) finally ran a study to confirm the results of Dr. Burzynski's treatment. The NIH treated the most dangerous and aggressive type of brain tumor (Glioblastoma) with a smaller dose than was recommended for that type of tumor. Dr. Burzynski had clearly instructed them on the correct protocol (with a clear dosing schedule), and they chose to treat with a protocol for a less aggressive tumor. This caused the results to be invalid because the NIH disregarded the protocol recommended by Dr. Burzynski, who had invented the medication and had run his own trials to show the results of the antineoplastin therapy at the appropriate and correct doses for each trial participant.

The NIH claimed the treatment was ineffective. The authorities seized Dr. Burzynskis' records and took him to court, charging him with shipping the medication across state lines. Parents were desperate to save their children, many of whom had been seriously damaged by the effects of chemotherapy and radiation. A tough battle was fought in court where many parents testified on behalf of their children, some of whom had passed away. People marched in the streets for the right of babies and toddlers with deadly brain tumors to receive this nontoxic and effective treatment. Dr. Burzynski was being persecuted. He owned the patents, and he owned a factory where the medication was manufactured.

The FDA director clearly stated that he would **not approve** a drug that was **not** produced by a major pharmaceutical company. They tried to take Dr. Burzynski's patents. They tried to discredit him. Lives of children were lost because of this bureaucracy. This man cures brain cancer in small children and gets attacked relentlessly and can't ship his medication over state lines. It is just maddening. I recommend you listen to the whole story. It's on YouTube.[214] I bought the DVD years ago with the story to support this amazing doctor. It is a story that should not be missed. Hopefully, this incredible medicine will be a mainstream treatment soon. As Dr. Burzynski says, "It is a new paradigm in medicine."[215] Anyone facing a diagnosis of cancer can visit the Burzynski Clinic in Houston, TX.

Intravenous Vitamin C Therapy

IV vitamin C therapy is currently used all over the world as a cancer treatment and it's widely available. My local integrative doctor offers it. It's typically $100–$150 per treatment and it's not covered by health insurance companies.

High doses of vitamin C given intravenously, usually 25–100 grams, have a pro-oxidative effect. That means that it promotes the formation of hydrogen peroxide within the tissues that accumulate the vitamin C. Cancer cells are particularly susceptible to damage by such reactive oxygen-containing compounds. Cancer cells cannot grow in the presence of oxygen. Intravenous vitamin C therapy has been used for over 25 years in the treatment of cancer.

The first physician to pioneer the use of vitamin C to cure diseases was Frederick R. Klenner, M.D. Starting in the early 1940s, Dr. Klenner, a pioneer in vitamin C research, successfully treated chicken pox, measles, mumps, tetanus, and polio with mega doses of vitamin C.

Conditions Successfully Treated with Intravenous Vitamin C Therapy

The following conditions were successfully treated by Dr. Klenner with aggressive vitamin C therapy.

Conditions Successfully Treated with Vitamin C Therapy			
Pneumonia	Corneal ulcer	Mononucleosis	Multiple sclerosis
Arthritis	Leukemia	Bladder infection	High cholesterol
Alcoholism	Glaucoma	Pancreatitis	Chronic fatigue
Diabetes	Heat stroke	Schizophrenia	Radiation burns
Hepatitis	Encephalitis	Atherosclerosis	Some cancers
Herpes simplex	Herpes zoster (shingles)	Complications of surgery	Burns and secondary infections

Conditions Successfully Treated with Vitamin C Therapy			
Ruptured intervertebral disc	Venomous bites (insects, snakes)	Heavy metal poisoning (mercury, lead)	Rocky Mountain spotted fever

Dr. Klenner used massive doses of vitamin C for over 40 years. He wrote 27 medical papers related to vitamin C treatment. Lendon H. Smith, M.D. documented a summary of the 27 papers Klenner published from the 1940s to the 1970s in the *Clinical Guide to the Use of Vitamin C*.[216]

Unfortunately, many medical experts chose to ignore his success in the research and treatment of disease. Dr. Klenner wrote: "Some physicians would stand by and see their patient die rather than use ascorbic acid (vitamin C) because in their finite minds it exists only as a vitamin." It still amazes and perplexes me how such *intelligent* beings can be so stubborn and resistant to life-saving treatments.

Vitamin C is remarkably safe even in enormously high doses. It does not cause kidney stones as some have claimed. In fact, vitamin C increases urine flow and helps lower the pH to prevent stones from forming. William J. McCormick, M.D. has used vitamin C since the late 1940s to *prevent and treat* kidney stones. Vitamin C does not significantly raise oxalate levels, and uric acid stones have never resulted from its use. Dr. Klenner said the ascorbic acid and kidney stone story is a myth.

Linus Pauling, rated the 16th most important scientist in history as of 2000, is probably the most well-renowned promoter of vitamin C research. Pauling was an American chemist, biochemist, peace activist, author, and educator. He was one of the most influential chemists in history and ranks among the most important scientists of the twentieth century. For his scientific work, Pauling was awarded the Nobel Prize in Chemistry in 1954.

In 1962, for his peace activism, he was awarded another Nobel Peace Prize. He was the only person to be awarded two unshared Nobel Prizes and one of five people to have won more than one Nobel Prize. He published more than 1200 papers and books, including many about the amazing benefits of vitamin C.[217]

At age 40, he was diagnosed with Bright's disease (a serious kidney disease). He lived to be 93 years old! He stayed well by eating a low-protein, salt-free diet, and vitamin supplements, including mega doses of vitamin C.

He wrote several articles and books about vitamin C, including, *Vitamin C and the Common Cold*; *Cancer and Vitamin C: A Discussion of the Nature, Causes, Prevention, and Treatment of Cancer with Special Reference to the Value of Vitamin C*; and *Healing Cancer: Complementary Vitamin & Drug Treatments*.

Pauling explained that one of the great misfortunes of human evolution was when our human ancestors lost their ability to manufacture vitamin C. He theorized that humans lost this ability during a time when people had a diet of vitamin-rich plants and didn't need to produce the vitamin themselves. Today, primates (including humans) are one of the few groups of animals that must get vitamin C through their diet. Due to that change in evolution, humans suffer from large deficiencies of vitamin C. He strongly recommended that people make up for this deficiency with daily doses of vitamin C **much greater than the 60 mg (RDA)**. Pauling said that the level of vitamin C that we consume should be on the same level as levels that other animals produce by themselves, which is typically **10–12 grams a day (10,000–12,000 mg)**. Pauling practiced what he preached, and gradually increased his daily doses of vitamin C from 3 grams in the 1960s to 18 grams. That's 18,000 mg. Do not be afraid to take too much vitamin C!

Vitamin C Prevents Cardiovascular Disease

Plaques build up in the blood vessels of people with atherosclerosis. Lipoprotein-a is a major component of that plaque. According to Linus Pauling, vitamin C is correlated with lipoprotein-a. Pauling published studies showing how lipoprotein-a substitutes for vitamin C, which strengthens blood vessel walls when people don't have enough vitamin C in their diet. Pauling strongly believed that high doses of **vitamin C can help prevent cardiovascular disease** by preventing the formation of lesions on blood vessel walls and decreasing the production of lipoprotein-a in the blood. Recent studies confirmed this finding! In addition, the combination of vitamin C and L-lysine have proven effective in removing plaques from arterial walls.[218]

Vitamin C Treatment for Various Cancers

Thanks to the work of Linus Pauling, intravenous vitamin C has been considered an integrative medical therapy for cancer since the 1970s. In fact, my primary physician offers it to cancer patients in his office. Studies in the 1970s and 1980s conducted by Linus Pauling, Ewan Cameron, and colleagues suggested that mega doses of vitamin C (10 grams per day intravenously for 10 days, followed by at least 10 grams per day by mouth indefinitely) helped to increase survival time and improve quality of life for terminal cancer patients.

Recent studies confirmed that high-dose intravenous vitamin C has the potential to be a potent anticancer agent.[219] In fact, many new studies have been published in various cancer journals including the *2009 Journal of the American Medical Association* (JAMA). There's now evidence that vitamin C provides protection from breast cancer. One study showed that women who supplemented with vitamin C for more than 10 years had a **42 percent reduced risk of developing breast cancer**. And higher vitamin C intake produced a **65 percent reduction in risk of cancer of the cervix**. Even **pancreatic cancer was shown**

to be 33 percent less likely in those with higher blood levels of vitamin C.

IV Vitamin C Kills Cancer Cells without Harming Normal Cells

Scientists at the University of Kansas found that when vitamin C is injected, it is absorbed into the body, and kills cancer cells without harming normal cells. The researchers injected vitamin C into human ovarian cancer cells in the lab, into mice, and into patients with advanced ovarian cancer. They found ovarian cancer cells responded to vitamin C treatment, but normal cells were unharmed. Administering IV vitamin C together with chemotherapy slowed tumor growth in mouse studies. They also observed that patients given vitamin C concurrently with chemotherapy reported less side effects from the chemotherapy.[220]

Thousands of People Died from Scurvy

Why isn't the amazing power of intravenous vitamin C known by everyone?

- First reason: It depends on who stands to profit.
- Second reason: There is an incredible amount of bias in the scientific community.

New discoveries and ideas are often rejected for years. Fresh fruit was said to cure scurvy by **1753**, but governments dismissed this fact for almost **100** years! Thousands of people died from scurvy during this time.

The 19th century doctor (Semmelweis) who first suggested health workers **wash their hands** between each patient to prevent infection was ostracized and disgraced. He died without knowing what an amazing impact he made.

Imagine the Number of Lives

Imagine the countless lives that were saved by preventing the spread of infection with the simple act of washing hands.

Now imagine how many lives would be saved by offering patients intravenous vitamin C therapy!

Over 60,000 People Died from Vioxx Medication

Sadly, it is not just close-mindedness. Pharmaceutical medications and vaccines are accepted and adopted into mainstream medicine more quickly and without the same type of bias applied to vitamins. New risky and dangerous drugs are often approved without long-term safety studies. Look at what happened with Vioxx. They discovered during clinical trials that many participants experienced cardiac arrest and many died. It was a significant number of deaths. The trial should have been canceled and the drug should not have been approved. Yet, they continued the trial and the drug was approved. Vioxx may have caused approximately 140,000 heart attacks resulting in an estimated 60,000 deaths, according to FDA investigator Graham.[221] Learning things like this is maddening, shocking, and disheartening. It drives me to teach safer ways to heal and to prevent disease.

Vitamin C Refused by Hospital

I tried to get vitamin C prescribed for my mother when she was ill with Covid-19 in a nursing home. I had an intense discussion with her "nurse practitioner" and finally got him to agree, but we did NOT agree on the dose. He would only agree to 500 mg two times a day, but I pushed for more and he agreed to 500 mg three times a day. That still was NOT enough to fight Covid-19, but I would have to settle. On the day she was to begin getting the vitamin C, she was moved from the nursing home to the hospital. I had the same discussion with the hospital doctor, and they told me they didn't have any vitamin C. I took a brand-new sealed bottle of vitamin C to the hospital. They *refused* to give it to her! There was absolutely no reason for them to refuse to give her vitamin C.

How to Get Vitamin C in the Hospital

Since then, I have learned that you can get intravenous vitamin C in the hospital if you prepare ahead of time. If you want the possibility of getting vitamin C administered intravenously to yourself or a loved one in the hospital, there are several steps you must take ahead of time, including getting a letter from your general practitioner and/or specialists you are working with. You can prepare yourself for their objections and their incorrect pronouncements of vitamin C not being an effective treatment. The complete strategy for working with hospitals to get vitamin C treatment, along with the research proving its effectiveness is available on Andrew Saul's website: Doctor Yourself.[222]

Will insurance company's cover the cost of intravenous vitamin C treatment? Not likely. Intravenous vitamin C treatments range in price from $125 to $160.

Detox Baths

Detox baths can help flush impurities from your body. Any detox bath you choose is fine but make sure you soak in hot water (not to burn you, but as hot as you can handle comfortably). The general rule is to soak for 20 to 40 minutes and hydrate well before and after.

If you do not have filtered water, add 1/2 cup of baking soda to neutralize the chemicals in the city water (1 to 2 tbsp for kids).

Essential Oils

You can add essential oils for aromatherapy, extra relaxation, and additional health benefits. Add five to ten drops of essential oils for adults, and three to five drops for kids. You can adjust as needed depending on the strength of your essential oils. With some brands, you may want to add more to really enjoy the aroma and the benefits. Some good choices include lavender, sandalwood, jasmine, frankincense, roman chamomile or rose.

Bentonite Clay

Bentonite clay is excellent at absorbing toxins. It's gentle enough to use with children.

- Add between 1–4 cups of bentonite clay (adults)
- Add between 1–2 cups of bentonite clay (kids)

You can blend the clay in a bowl of warm water first and then pour it into the tub. While you soak in the warm water, the clay goes to work absorbing the toxins from your skin. The clay particles adsorb the toxins into their own molecules because toxins have positive electrons and clay particles have negative electrons. Therefore, the clay draws the toxins out.

Epsom Salt

- Add two cups of Epsom salt and 5–10 drops of essentials oils (adults)
- Add 1/2 cup of Epsom salt and 3–5 drops of essentials oils (kids)

Sea Salt or Himalayan Salt

- Add two cups of sea salt or Himalayan salt (adults)
- Add 1/2 cup to one cup of sea salt or Himalayan salt (kids)

Strong All-Purpose Detox Bath

- Add two cups of sea salt or Himalayan salt
- Add two cups of baking soda
- Add one cup of 20 Mule Team borax powder

Recommendations

This chapter covered many effective and proven cancer-fighting gems. These are preventative natural treatments that can extend your life. Aside from periodic detoxification, try to ensure that you are consuming plenty of antioxidants, fruits and vegetables, clean protein, fermented foods, and clean water. Also make sure you maintain an optimal vitamin D level (60-80). Several studies have found a beneficial impact of vitamin D in reducing cancer risk, treating cancer, and reducing the number of cancer deaths.[223]

CHAPTER 15

Epigenetics: Genes are not Destiny

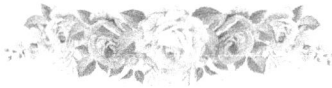

"The more I learn, the less I realize I know."
– Socrates

Many people think they are destined to suffer the same diseases as their family members. However, the study of epigenetics teaches us that genes play an important role in our health, but that our behavior, environment, and habits can change the way our genes work. The study of "epigenetics" has shown that your genes are not your destiny. Your genes play a part in your risk for developing disease, but you can change your epigenetics with your life choices.

Genetic mutations or damaged genes are like weak links in a chain that affect your likelihood of having conditions such as thyroid disease, autoimmune disease, ADHD, cancer, and even weight gain. If a link is stressed or damaged enough times, it can break and lead to a state of disease. These weaknesses can be strengthened.

Dr. Ben Lynch, author of *Dirty Genes,* is a leading expert in the field of epigenetics. He teaches about genetic variations and how you can reduce your risk of disease by "cleaning your genes." A gene that is "dirty" is not functioning correctly either because you were born with mutations or because their function is impaired by diet and lifestyle choices, environmental contaminants, or mental health.

The genetic predisposition for autoimmunity is 30 percent. In contrast, *environmental* factors trigger an autoimmune response 70 percent of the time. While environmental triggers are a substantially bigger threat, gene mutations and damage should still be addressed because you cannot detox efficiently if you are not "methylating" or eliminating toxins effectively.

Gene mutations came onto my radar in 2012 when a doctor tested me for the MTHFR gene. It was a bit shocking initially to receive a lab result telling me I had mutated genes. I remember feeling upset and telling a close friend, "I'm a mutant!" However, soon I learned that everyone has gene mutations. Dr. Jerk did not explain it very well, so I started digging in and found Dr. Ben Lynch online. I later attended a summit and listened to several presentations about epigenetics and gene mutations. It was at this summit where I was blown away by one speaker, Sterling Hill Erdei. She spoke quickly and passionately, and she conveyed information masterfully. I took notes furiously. I learned from her how to upload the Excel file I received from 23andMe to a website and generate a report that shows all your genes in a color-coded chart. If you are a 23andMe customer, you already have access to the Excel spreadsheet. If not, you can either go through 23andMe or you can ask your doctor to run genetic testing.

Sterling Hill Erdei is the founder of MTHFR Support.[224] She shares her compelling story on their website. She was a very successful businesswoman, but she became ill with clotting issues, and she lost everything because all the physicians she sought help from did not understand her condition. Her health continued to deteriorate until she found the alternative medicine community. She learned that the cause of her clotting issues was related to the sulfation and methylation cycle. After she recovered and got her life back, her new mission was to spread the word about epigenetics and nutrigenomics. Nutrigenomics is the study of the interaction of nutrition and genes, especially in relation to the prevention or treatment of disease.

This is a complex subject. If you get your gene reports, you can get overwhelmed and just put it down for later, which is what I did for several years. I printed out two huge reports. I looked up my gene variants and learned the basics. I took the reports to three different doctors, and they gave them a glance and didn't offer any advice whatsoever. That was discouraging. I was alone in my effort to figure out what I should do.

Dr. Lynch provides expert guidance is this area. Epigenetics is the science of understanding how your genes are expressed and how you can use diet, supplements, environment, and lifestyle to help you to prevent disease that you are genetically predisposed to. When you understand what your genes need, you can choose a diet and lifestyle that gives you a higher chance of living your life disease-free. The goal is to feel happy, healthy, and energetic. It's not easy. Dr. Lynch warns that if you continue to eat poorly, sleep poorly, and deprive your body of the nutrients that it needs to thrive, you will be more prone to depression, anxiety, ADHD, insomnia, heart disease, obesity, food cravings, fatigue, addictions, and many other disorders.

s

Methylation is Critical to your Health

Methylation is a process that takes place approximately one billion times per second and affects nearly every essential process in the body. It is important for energy levels, hormone balance, detoxification, mental health, and more. In general terms, methylation and demethylation is the transfer of methyl groups, which are structures of one carbon and three hydrogen molecules (CH3), to and from many different biological compounds in the body. These compounds include proteins, enzymes, hormones, and others. They must be methylated to work correctly and to create other substances that your body needs. When it comes to detoxification, if your methylation process is not working well, it is like there is a cog in the machine. Something is essentially blocking your body from letting go of, or excreting toxins such as heavy metals and pesticides. These harmful toxins increase your risk for cancer and other diseases. It also causes your liver to hold on to harmful fats which increase your tendency to gain weight and hold on to weight.

MTHFR Genetic Mutations (Variants)

Some sources say 30–40 percent of people have MTHFR gene mutations. Up to 55 percent of the European population have MTHFR gene mutations.[225] I am one of them. My children both have them.

You can have either one or two mutations (or neither) on each MTHFR gene. These mutations are called variants. A variant is a part of a gene's DNA that is different, or varies, from one person to another. If you have:

- One variant, it is "heterozygous." This is less likely to contribute to health issues.
- Two variants, it is "homozygous." This may lead to more serious problems.

There are two variants that can occur on the MTHFR gene: C677T and A1298C. Refer to the bottom two rows of the following chart.

rs1650697	DHFR/MSH T-473A	G	GG	+/+
rs1050829	G6PD A376G - Class I	C	TT	-/-
rs5030868	G6PD S219F - Class II	A	GG	-/-
rs1050828	G6PD V98M - Class III	T	CC	-/-
rs1050450	GPX1 200 Pro>Leu	A	GG	-/-
rs1138272	GSTP1 A114V	T	CT	+/-
rs1695	GSTP1 I105V	G	AG	+/-
rs6323	MAOA R297R/G492T/T941G	T	GT	+/-
rs1137070	MAOA T1011C/1460C	C	CT	+/-
rs1799836	MAOB A118723G	C	TT	-/-
rs2236225	MTHFD1 R635Q	A	GG	-/-
rs1801131	MTHFR A1298C	G	GT	+/-
rs1801133	MTHFR C677T	A	AG	+/-

Sample from Genome Report

Many people with MTHFR gene mutations have problems with methylation. One serious problem associated with the MTHFR gene mutation is the reduced ability to convert folate into methylene tetrahydrofolate reductase (MTHFR), which is the enzyme needed for many parts of the methylation process.

The MTHFR enzyme plays an important role in processing amino acids. It helps convert homocysteine to methionine. MTHFR deficiency, or genetic variations in the MTHFR gene, can lead to high levels of homocysteine in the blood and low levels of folate and other vitamins.

Epigenetics Research

The process of turning genes on and off is called epigenetics. These changes do not change the DNA sequence. They affect how the genes are expressed. Factors that affect the genes being turned on or off are development (in utero or childhood), environmental chemicals, drugs, pharmaceuticals, aging, and diet.

Recent scientific research has demonstrated that the epigenome can change in response to the environment throughout the lifetime of the person. In one recent experiment with mice, dirty genes were disabled! Some of the mothers were given methyl donors and some were not. Methyl donors are nutrients that support methylation, such as methylated B12 and folate. The dirty genes of the mice that received the methyl donors were effectively turned off and were expressed differently in their offspring![226] **This indicates it's possible to transform your genetic destiny** by using a combination of diet, supplements, sleep, stress relief, and reduced exposure to environmental toxins. That is powerful!

Therefore, you are **not** doomed to inherit every disease of your family or ancestors. I've heard people speak helplessly about conditions such as psoriasis, tremors, cancer, Alzheimer's, and more. It's sad to see people so resigned with that "I give up" attitude. In my experience, many of them were not even open to listening to how to prevent the "hereditary" diseases. When I start talking about epigenetics to some folks and explain that only a small percentage of diseases are truly genetic, they sometimes don't believe me. The old model of thought is very ingrained in some people, while others are very open to it. I appreciate being able to share this hopeful information with people.

With the right tools, you can reduce your chances of inheriting diseases, such as anxiety, ADHD, birth defects, cancer, dementia, depression, heart disease, insomnia, and obesity. If you can identify your dirty genes, you can develop a protocol to scrub them clean and replace disease with health which enables you to reach your genetic potential! If you have adult children that are willing to learn about this, you can improve your chances of having healthy grandchildren! How wonderful is that?

Recommendations

Although this is a complex topic, an easy way to get started is to supplement with methyl B12 (methylcobalamin) and methylfolate. The methylated form of these two B vitamins help your body to methylate better. They are called *methyl donors*. Improving your methylation helps you to detox better and create health rather than illness.

- Vitamin B12—Methylcobalamin—the metabolically active form of B12
- Folate—Methylfolate 5-MTHF (L-Methylfolate)—the metabolically active form of folic acid

You can improve your genetic health with good sleep, exercise, regular detoxification, and a nutritious diet and supplementation program. Also, remember from Chapter 13, that glutathione and medicinal mushrooms help to repair and support production of DNA. I also recommend getting your genetic testing done if you haven't already. There are many resources available to help you understand how your specific genes affect your health. It's very interesting to learn how your genes influence not only your risks of disease, but your behavior, appearance, taste preferences, test-taking skills, and more. If you learn which of your genes have variants, you can take positive steps toward maintaining your health and preventing future disease. For more information, see Dr. Ben Lynch's book, Dirty Genes, and his website.[227]

CHAPTER 16

Advanced Holistic Treatments

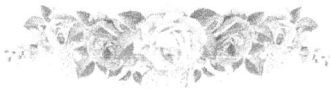

"You can learn new things at any time in your life if you're willing to be a beginner. If you actually learn to like being a beginner, the whole world opens up to you."
– Barbara Sher

If you have Hashimoto's disease or virtually any other autoimmune disease, there are a multitude of alternative treatments that you can try. Some are expensive, while some can be done in your home at a low cost. The following treatments can be helpful for your immunity, thyroid health, emotional health, and overall well-being.

Red Light Therapy

Red light therapy (RLT) is a form of low-level laser light therapy (LLLT) and is also known as photo biomodulation or cold laser therapy. It is perfectly safe and very therapeutic.

Red light therapy devices emit low-intensity lasers or light-emitting diodes (LED lights) at specific wavelengths to promote healing. These devices are available for at-home use as hand-held wands and massage devices, neck wraps, body wraps, face masks, or belts, and large metal light panel boxes in a range of sizes. They are also available in spas and chiropractor offices.

Many of us with Hashimoto's suffer from joint pain and stiffness, and many of us start to develop arthritis as we get older. This is a painful and difficult problem to deal with. I have had days when everything hurt but fortunately not all at once! I've had pain in my hands, feet, ankles, knees, lower back, shoulders, upper back, and neck. I invested in a Platinum LED red light therapy panel, and it really does help to relieve pain and stiffness right away. I also have red light devices in the form of a neck collar, a wrap for my lower back, and a hand-held massager.

Numerous research studies have found RLT to be beneficial for pain and inflammation. It can reduce pain when used consistently at a recommended dose. It has been shown to be effective for spasms, pain, and inflammation providing both short- and long-term relief. Some people experience pain relief immediately and some notice relief over hours or days. RLT helps with inflammation-related chronic health issues, including tendonitis, obesity, rheumatoid arthritis, osteoarthritis, psoriasis, and autoimmune thyroiditis.[228]

In addition to helping with pain and inflammation, red light therapy has many other benefits. First and foremost, **red light therapy has been shown to improve thyroid function!** In one study, where patients with hypothyroidism caused by Hashimoto's received 10 sessions of LLLT, the treatment resulted in reduced TPOAb (thyroid antibody) levels and less need for levothyroxine (T4) treatment. In fact, during a nine-month follow-up, **47** percent of patients no longer needed levothyroxine.[229]

Additional benefits of LLLT include:

- Promotes wound healing, tissue repair, and tissue regeneration
- Supports collagen production and thus helps prevent skin aging
- Stimulates mitochondrial health
- Supports hair growth
- Improves circadian rhythm and sleep
- Reduces inflammation and pain

Many recent LLLT research studies have shown promising results for a wide variety of health problems, including:

- Neurological issues (including stroke and traumatic brain injuries)[230]
- Skin conditions (including scars, acne, wrinkles, burns, herpes lesions, and psoriasis)[231]
- Orthodontic issues (including tooth movement acceleration and pain relief)[232]
- Hair loss due to androgenetic alopecia[233]
- Fibromyalgia symptoms (including musculoskeletal or neuropathic pain, fatigue, and depression)[234]

LLLT also helps with blood flow and joint inflammation by triggering the relaxation of smooth muscles in the blood vessels, which allows more oxygen into the affected cells. In a study published in 2015, researchers suggested that **orthopedic surgeons can improve outcomes and reduce adverse events by using LLLT.**[235] I had shoulder surgery in 2020. Neither my shoulder surgeon, nor about eight different physical therapists, were astute enough to offer or recommend LLLT to their patients. It could have helped my tissue to regenerate and heal faster and it could have reduced my pain and inflammation, especially during the 10-month period of grueling physical therapy. Change is so slow in the medical community. Thankfully I am benefitting from it now, and I highly recommend it. It's affordable and it works.

Frequency Healing

There are a variety of technologies that use frequencies to treat illnesses. This technology is nothing new. It was developed almost 100 years ago. I personally own a Rife machine, and a scalar energy machine. I also go to a center that has an EESystem™.

The Energy Enhancement System™ generates multiple bio-active life enhancing energy fields, including "scalar waves" which can allow cell regeneration, improve immune function, provide relief from pain, detoxify the body, elevate moods, and assist in balancing right and left hemispheres of the brain to increase energy levels. I have had some significant gains in my life from this technology, including a complete recovery from plantar fasciitis and a heel spur which caused several years of terrible foot pain.

Rife machines use the principles of Royal Rife, who was a brilliant scientist and inventor who lived during the last century. He discovered that micro-organisms can be destroyed using frequencies. He performed thousands of experiments, each demonstrating that cancer has a viral cause, and that damaging this virus almost always resulted in a cure. Rife machines made national news in the U.S. in the 1930s after gaining support from a group of 44 doctors who announced the "end of all disease." Soon thereafter, powerful business interests apparently threatened the doctors and the inventor (who fled to Mexico) and the information was buried. The early Rife machines and documentation were destroyed. However, in recent years, there has been renewed interest and a variety of these machines are now widely available.

I personally used my Rife machine to lower my blood sugar dramatically (from 210 to 125) on the first attempt, and the next day, after running it again, it went down to 112. I have also used it for many other health issues. The possibilities are virtually endless.

Acupuncture

Acupuncturists insert thin needles into specific points on the body to help balance the body's energy, which is thought to reduce or resolve symptoms of illness including pain and anxiety.

I had a series of acupuncture treatments from four different acupuncturists over the years. I found it to be deeply relaxing, but it didn't help with my shoulder pain or thyroid, and I didn't notice any long-term results. I am not saying it doesn't work. I know other people have great results. It just didn't work for me after multiple attempts, so I did not consider it cost-effective in my case.

Emotional Therapy

Emotional wellness is a key aspect of overall health and well-being. Emotional wellness helps you to:

- Be more aware of your emotional reactions, thoughts, and behaviors
- Manage stress and emotions in a healthy way
- Bounce back from emotionally traumatic experiences and become more resilient
- Communicate effectively, build healthy relationships, and maintain positive connections with others
- Build healthy self-esteem, feel good about yourself, and develop a positive self-image

Emotional wellness helps you to lead a happy, healthy, and fulfilling life. Not everyone gets emotionally well the same way.

Some people find it therapeutic to talk through their issues and come to conclusions together with another person, whether it be a friend, family member, or professional counselor.

I personally did not find it beneficial to talk through my traumas and problems. I visited a traditional talk therapist twice. All they did was let me talk, while they took notes. Neither of them offered one single word of advice or direction. I can talk to myself for free! I don't have the patience for that long and expensive approach. It's just not for me.

Spiritual therapists with intuitive abilities are my preferred option. I have consulted with several people with special abilities that enabled them to get to the root cause of my issues more quickly. I am intuitive myself and I naturally gravitate toward people that I vibe with. These practitioners were also interactive and communicated both ways, instead of just sitting there writing on a pad. I also have spiritual practices that help me to soothe my emotions.

Try different things and go with what makes you most comfortable. You don't need approval from *anyone*. Do what works for you.

Massage Therapy

Count yourself lucky if you have a loved one to provide you with massage therapy. Massage can be for relaxation or pleasure, but therapeutic massage helps to reduce stiffness, pain, stress, and inflammation. It helps your body release toxins by stimulating circulation and lymphatic drainage which promotes detoxification. While massage is an extra expense, I do my own nails, make my own coffee, and cook for myself most of the time. For me, spending money on something that helps me feel better is worth it. I found a wonderful therapist that I trust with my care. It's important to find someone that you can talk to and communicate comfortably when you are in pain and someone that is skilled in therapeutic techniques.

Essential Oils

Initially, I thought essential oils smelled good and were helpful for relaxation and even headaches. As I dug deeper, I learned more about the benefits of essential oils. They can be very useful in medicinal ways, especially when you use 100 percent pure and therapeutic grade oils. I started to use high quality essential oils including lavender, tea tree, peppermint, orange, frankincense, myrrh, ylang ylang, lemongrass, and cinnamon, and I had excellent results. I started to make deodorant, sprays, rollers, and ointments and give them to friends and family. My mom and my friends love my lavender deodorant and antibiotic ointment. A few years later, I started a small business and called it "Indigo Healing Oils." I created a product line of crystal-infused essential oil products which I sold online and at local events.

Recently, I decided to close my online store because it's too expensive to maintain the website, buy insurance, create content for social media, and pay for marketing. It is very difficult to be profitable especially with so many competing companies. I am definitely a dreamer, and I am a positive thinker to a fault. I didn't realize how hard it is to market, sell, and compete in the marketplace.

However, it makes me happy when I work with the essential oils, probably because so many of them reduce stress and boost your mood. I enjoy creating things like body butter, scrubs, hair growth oil, pain cream, soaps, and more. Relieving pain is one of my favorite aspects of working with essential oils. The anti-inflammatory effects are very effective. I use my cinnamon frankincense pain cream often when I have pain. I continue to make products in small batches when time allows.

I developed many well-researched blends. In fact, my Thyroid Balance product contains some of the best essential oils for the thyroid. I roll it directly on my neck for my thyroid. It contains a specially formulated blend of 100 percent pure essential oils, and it is infused with the lapis lazuli crystal. It smells wonderful and it contains the following ingredients: Fractionated coconut oil, frankincense, lemongrass, myrrh, peppermint, geranium, clary sage, and clove.

The benefits of the essential oils in Indigo Thyroid Balance are described below.

Frankincense: Promotes healthy immune and endocrine health and decreases inflammation. Frankincense can also balance hormone levels, reduce stress, and help you to sleep better at night.

Lemongrass: Can help with inflammation, headaches, and digestive upset associated with an under-active thyroid. It also has soothing and calming effects on the mind, relieving tension and anxiety.

Myrrh: Studies show that myrrh has anti-inflammatory, antioxidant, and immunoprotective properties and can be beneficial for the immune system. *Life Extension* published an article that mentioned that myrrh may help with the conversion of T4 to T3.[236] Another study showed that myrrh essential oil can modulate both Th1 and Th2 cytokines.[237] Anecdotal evidence has shown that rubbing a few drops of myrrh essential oil around the thyroid gland may be able to help benefit thyroid health, and in some cases reduce a goiter.

Peppermint: Can help reduce fatigue, depression, anxiety, brain fog, headaches, and digestive issues associated with an underactive thyroid. Peppermint also helps to stimulate the thyroid.

Geranium: Is anti-inflammatory and helps to stimulate the production of thyroid hormones.

Clary sage: Helps reduce stress and high cortisol levels, improve cognitive function, and help with digestion and hair loss.

Clove: Helps to improve thyroid function, balance hormones, and calm down inflammation.

Crystal properties: Lapis Lazuli is beneficial to the throat, larynx, and vocal cords, and helps regulate the endocrine and thyroid glands. The throat chakra is represented by blue, and it is the voice of the body. Blue crystal energy helps to unblock and balance the throat chakra. When in balance, it allows for the expression of what we think and what we feel. We can communicate our ideas, beliefs, and emotions.

Warning: As mentioned in Chapter 9, essential oils must be diluted before you apply them to your skin. You should use a prepared blend or add a few drops of a pure essential oil to a quality carrier oil. Also, avoid oral ingestion (swallowing) of essential oils. It can be dangerous. If you want to take essential oils internally, you should work with a qualified aromatherapist, herbalist, or doctor.

Bach Flower Essences

I probably would not have used flower essences as much as I did if it were not for a friend that talked about them all the time. Years ago, I was angry with a guy I used to date when he stood me up for the umpteenth time!! I was so angry and I started to feel a sharp pain on the right side of my chest. My friend said that I should rub holly flower essence directly on my chest and I did. The pain disappeared instantly. I was impressed and started to use a few of the essences for various emotional issues. I have had experiences where the essences worked instantly or over time, or where the effect was more subtle or not noticeable at all. I now have the entire set of Bach flower essences so that I can make custom formulas.

It's very interesting to learn about how the essence of a flower can affect your spiritual body. Your body is surrounded by your energy force, light body, aura, or whatever you want to call it. We are all made of energy and that extends beyond our physical body. That's why you can feel positive or negative energy or "vibes" from people.

What is more interesting is that each emotion maps to parts of your body. Holly for example, maps to the right chest area as well as a few other areas. Holly helps with anger and resentment in relation to the heart. Sweet chestnut is helpful with mental anguish. I was feeling anguish for a time, and I developed an angry red eczema patch about three inches in diameter on the back of my upper thigh. It was very itchy and irritating. I tried many things including eczema, antifungal, and antibiotic ointments. Finally, I decided to look up the affected body part in my *Bach Flower Body Map* book and it mapped to sweet chestnut (mental anguish). I started taking two to three drops by mouth per day, and it quickly disappeared and never came back. That was an impressive result.

There are flower essences that address all kinds of emotions, including guilt, despair, hopelessness, fear of known things, fear of unknown things, addiction, panic, exhaustion, lack of confidence, and more. There are thirty-eight Bach flower essences. The Rescue Remedy product is very popular and contains five flower essences that help people that feel intense fear, anxiety, shock, or panic.

There are many resources online, but these two books are most helpful to me: *New Bach Flower Body Maps* by Dietmar Kramer, and *The Encyclopedia of Bach Flower Therapy* by Mechthild Scheffer.

Hyperbaric Oxygen Therapy

Hyperbaric Oxygen Therapy (HBOT) can be helpful for many health conditions, including **autoimmune disease**, dementia, diabetes, cancer, Lyme disease, mold toxicity, migraines, wounds, autism, traumatic brain injuries, strokes, burns, and more. It oxygenates body tissue which helps reduce inflammation, heal infections, and repair damaged tissues. HBOT floods the body with oxygen. In one hour of HBOT treatment, the body takes in about 2.4 pounds of oxygen. This increases the oxygen level in the tissues by 10 to 15 times more than the amount you get with normal breathing.

Increased oxygen into the body can provide the following benefits:

- Stimulates growth of new blood vessels and capillaries
- Helps with simple wound healing
- Helps fight infections
- Reduces swelling and inflammation
- Improves cognitive function
- Stimulates brain cells and improves cerebral blood flow

HBOT helps autoimmune diseases as follows:

- Reduces systemic inflammation and inflammation at the cellular level
- Lowers c-reactive proteins and cytokine levels (markers of chronic inflammation)
- Rebalances the immune system, increases energy levels, and improves brain function
- May influence our epigenetics, turning off inflammatory genes and turning on growth and repair genes
- Immune modulating: calms the immune system to prevent self-attacking

As more people have discovered its health benefits, hyperbaric oxygen therapy has become more widely available. I have read four books on oxygen therapy, and I find it very hopeful. I personally went for a few treatments. It was relaxing and helped my energy level. I didn't continue simply because of the cost and the long drive to the facility. I wish mainstream medicine would prescribe and cover it for the many conditions it can help. Prescribing HBOT therapy could potentially help millions of people but it is only FDA-approved for about 12 conditions and they do not include any autoimmune diseases. Many studies have shown benefits beyond this list.

Stem Cell Therapy

I believe there is great promise in stem cell therapy. However, it is very expensive. I paid $10,000 for stem cell surgery for my shoulder when I had a torn bicep, labral, and rotator cuff, and it didn't work at ALL. In addition to my shoulder, my neck and knees were treated. After that failed, I had to have orthopedic surgery. Some say that celebrities that maintain their youth are privy to expensive stem cell treatments. That might be true. I know it works for many people. This particular treatment just didn't work for me.

I was told later by a doctor that provides stem cell treatments, that as you get older, your stem cells are less viable. Of course, Dr. StemCellFail did not mention that concern. He didn't suggest we use exosomes or anything other than my own stem cells. Did my cells fail me? Did they harvest them incorrectly? He did not discuss the other available options with me. Some say it is more effective to use exosomes, which are stem cells taken from umbilical cord blood.

There is a lot of research going on in this area and many treatments are available. In 2020, a study was published that showed immune modulating benefits for autoimmune disease using adult stem cells.[238] Mesenchymal stem cells (MSCs) are derived from adult tissues and can be safely harvested and used for stem cell therapy. MSCs can boost immune activity, promoting inflammation when the immune system is underactive. MSCs can also restrain inflammation when the immune system is overactive and attacking. MSCs have been successfully used to treat diabetes[239], cardiovascular disease[240], and autoimmune diseases.[241]

A new and promising treatment currently in clinical trials is the Sernova Cell Pouch. This Therapy is showing promising results in trials for **regenerating thyroid tissue after a total thyroidectomy**. It is also being studied to treat other diseases including autoimmune disease and diabetes.[242] Sernova's Cell Pouch is an implantable device that when used in combination with immune-protected therapeutic cells, offers protection from immune system attacks.

Muscle Testing

It seems strange at first, but I think there is something to muscle testing. Is it 100 percent scientifically accurate? I doubt it! But neither is your doctor's advice. He is just practicing after all! My holistic dentist used muscle testing on my son to determine which filling material to use for him. He made my skeptical son a believer because of the way his arm weakened when presented with certain materials. You can do it on yourself by practicing what some people call the sway technique.

You can assess if an item is good for you as follows. Stand up and hold a supplement or medication up to your chest. Relax your body and don't think too much. Don't fight the sway. Notice if your body naturally sways forward or backward. If you sway forward, that is a positive result. If you sway backwards, it's not for you. You can also have another person muscle test you. You hold the item with one hand against your chest and hold your other arm straight out to your side. The other person tries to push it down while you resist. If the arm weakens easily, it's not for you. If the arm stays strong, it may be helpful.

CHAPTER 17

Spiritual Health and Healing

"Among other things, neuroplasticity means that emotions such as happiness and compassion can be cultivated in much the same way that a person can learn through repetition to play golf and basketball or master a musical instrument, and that such practice changes the activity and physical aspects of specific brain areas."
— Dr. Andrew Weil

For me, spiritual healing goes hand in hand with the physical. The connection between body, mind, and spirit is well established. Weakness in one of these areas can affect the others.

Connect with Your Higher Self

I believe that your higher self and your ancestors want to communicate with you and guide you to be happy, healthy, and the best version of you possible. By tapping into your higher self, you can put yourself on a path of growth, peace, and abundance that not only benefits you, but the people around you as well. Of course, this applies to animals as well. It is clear that animals gravitate toward people with gentle positive energy. In turn, connecting with animals and nature feeds your soul and benefits your health. In fact, studies show that people that spend time in nature and those who own pets benefit from more balanced blood pressure and less depression.

Connecting to your higher self can lead to many advantages, such as:

- Higher sense of intuition
- Guidance received through dreams
- Recognizing signs that we receive from our ancestors and spirit guides
- Chance encounters with special people
- Coincidentally finding information or music that is just what you need
- Tuning in to people that really need you
- Learning to love yourself and others more deeply
- Staying true to yourself and speaking honestly
- Unplugging from the world—you're no longer worried about those in power, media, government, or business. You acknowledge their hidden agendas and understand that there is so much more to life.

Celestial Inspiration

I think a lot of us are naturally drawn to look at the moon and the stars and wonder about our connection with the universe. I have had several dreams where I was flying through the stars in the universe, and two dreams where I saw beautiful star-filled constellations in the sky. I receive messages through my dreams on a regular basis and you can too if you pay attention and try to interpret symbols that you see in your dreams.

I enjoy drawing inspiration from books, including the bible, and books about personal growth, ancient civilizations, near-death experiences, angels, and spiritual connection. What is life? What happens after death? It's a very personal experience. My family was separated by religion, and it caused a lot of emotional trauma and lost love and lost time for many of my family members. I grew up and decided to be more open and accepting. People can choose whatever religion they want, but I do not believe they have the right to judge other people's faith. As someone raised in a strict Christian religion, I was taught not to even enter another church but after growing up and exploring various religions and topics, I found my own path. I started to experience a "flow" and many signs and confirmations happened along the way to affirm I was on the right track. I am still a Christian. That is something my mother and I shared, and that will never change. I accept Jesus Christ as my Lord and Savior.

I believe that we all have a guardian angel and other spirit guides that include our ancestors. I know that I receive guidance from my ancestors. That feeling of connection is soothing and affirming. I love learning about the angels. I have received signs from angels on several occasions that affirmed what I was learning about.

I dream with my mother every so often and I am always so happy to see her. I recently had a beautiful dream with her where she was sitting on my front porch with me and I just held her in both of my arms and smiled a mile wide and told her how much I loved her and missed her, and then I had one arm around her as we talked. I remember telling her about the chicken tortilla soup that I made. It was so real and I woke up feeling joyful and melancholy at the same time. She may not be here with me in person but we will always be connected in spirit. I think if you remain open and pay attention, you receive signs that keep you connected.

4:7:8 Breathing Exercise to Reduce Stress

This breathing exercise is a natural tranquilizer for your nervous system. It works better with time, repetition, and practice, unlike tranquilizing drugs, which are often effective at first but then lose power over time. Use this method to relax, fall asleep or whenever you are tense or upset.

Sit up straight if possible.

1. Exhale completely through your mouth, making a whoosh sound.
2. Close your mouth and inhale quietly through your nose to a mental count of 4.
3. Hold your breath for a count of 7.
4. Exhale completely through your mouth, making a whoosh sound to a count of 8.
5. This is one breath. Now inhale again and repeat the cycle three more times for a total of four breaths. Later you can increase to eight breaths if you want.

Do this exercise at least twice a day. If you feel a little lightheaded when you first breathe this way, do not worry. It will pass.

Reiki Energy Work

I believe Reiki has real benefits, especially for those that are open to energy work. I don't have a lot of personal experience with it. I completed a level one Reiki certification, but I didn't pursue it any further. However, one day I had a psychic reading with a woman I was becoming friends with. She told me she had a headache and I immediately felt compassion for her. Without telling her anything, I started sending her healing energy to help her with her headache. I visualized light traveling to her with the intention of helping her headache. Just a couple minutes later, she asked me if I was sending her energy! She felt it and her headache went away. I was amazed. It might sound strange, but it is real. Some people claim they don't believe what they can't see, but they believe in Wi-Fi right? When's the last time you *saw* Wi-Fi?

Forgiveness

Forgiveness is a powerful tool that can help you release anger and resentment towards those who have harmed you or your family. It can be challenging to forgive someone who has caused you pain, but it is important to remember that forgiveness does not mean that you condone their behavior. Instead, it is about freeing yourself from the burden of anger and bitterness.

One of the most powerful scriptures about forgiveness is found in Matthew 6:14-15, where Jesus teaches, "For if you forgive others their trespasses, your heavenly Father will also forgive you, but if you do not forgive others their trespasses, neither will your Father forgive your trespasses." This passage reminds us that forgiveness is not just a good thing to do, but it is necessary for our own spiritual well-being.

Forgive all those who have wronged you (in your heart). Try to find some compassion for them. Do it for yourself to lighten your load and make your energy brighter and more positive.

Prayers

Prayers are another way to connect and find peace, or just express yourself talking to God. Having faith in a higher power is a healthy way to connect, no matter what your belief system.

CHAPTER 18

Imperfection and Self Sabotage

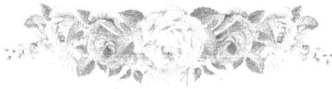

"Falling down is not a failure. Failure comes when you stay where you have fallen."
– Socrates

Although I am a board-certified drugless practitioner with multiple certifications, I do not follow a rigid health regimen with flawless dedication. I would like to, and I admire others that do. It took me a long time to realize why I have such difficulty with 'stick-to-itive-ness'—which is defined as dogged perseverance, or tenacity. It is not a weak will. I think it is due to my brain chemistry and my spiritual nature as a sensitive, intuitive triple Gemini. As a child, I was a free spirit and I explored nature. I often played alone in the woods without a care in the world. I was eternally curious. I was open to experiencing everything I could in life. I played all kinds of sports (football, volleyball, trackball, badminton, soccer, softball, baseball, and kickball). I skateboarded, biked, roller skated, ice skated, sledded, climbed trees, swam, made doll clothes and all kinds of crafts. You name it. I did it. I also helped my mom clean the house, the yard, and the car. I attended religious meetings with my mom three times a week. I went to school and got good grades without trying too hard. I got my homework done fast so I could play.

I was diagnosed as a child with hyperactivity and I still have it as an adult. You could call this a problem. It has its pluses and minuses. It is hard to stay tidy and organized. It's hard to be on time. My mind is always busy. I've worked very hard to improve my communication skills and time management. I'm often misunderstood, but there is a positive side. Essentially, I have severe ADHD which I sometimes call "Attention Dialed to a Higher Dimension." Most people with ADHD learn coping mechanisms, but it does not go away. You just learn how to manage. I may not be the most organized person and I have a lot going on, including many projects, but I accomplish a lot, and I hold on tightly to my dreams.

As an adult, I have the capability to hyperfocus and accomplish things quickly. I am very motivated to learn because I discovered my passion early in my twenties. Due to synchronicity, I naturally encounter people, books, summits, conferences, and courses related to my passions. I am constantly learning and gathering information, drawing inspiration, and experimenting with new foods, supplements, ideas, and treatments. However, due to my mercurial nature, I find it difficult to stick to a program for a long period of time. I adjust my regimen all the time. I do the best I can every day. Every day, I wake up with my goals for the day in mind. I don't always meet those goals, but I accomplish at least some of them and I don't beat myself up if I miss something. I feel confident that I will continue to lose weight and heal the issues that I still face. I never give up! I have come so far. I feel exponentially better than I did before and that gives me faith, contentment, and calmness. I feel like I can heal just about anything! People that can pick up a new diet or program and just go for it and be successful impress me. If you are one of them, congratulations. I admire you! If you are like the rest of us who have trouble deciding on and then following a certain regimen, be patient with yourself and stay positive. Just don't give up. I'm sure many of you experience overwhelm. At times, I get overwhelmed with so many pressures, resulting in a lapse of self-care. Sometimes, I get so wrapped up in things, that I forget about some supplements and indulge in the wrong foods. It happens to everyone.

We all experience fluctuations in our energy and motivation. No one is perfect even if they try to portray it on the outside. For many of us, stress and emotional upset can throw us off track. Every day is a new opportunity to do your best. Start fresh each day, eat as cleanly as possible, and detox from time to time. Plan your meals and nutritional drinks ahead of time as much as possible.

It's easy to get overwhelmed and throw your hands up and just eat whatever. I get it. When I received my first set of food allergy results on an IGG test, every food I loved was listed in red. This indicated that my body was producing antibodies to those foods. Dr. Jerk indicated that I was allergic to all those foods. I could not imagine how I would handle cutting out ALL those foods. I also wondered nervously what the heck I would eat! It turned out that test result was inaccurate. All the foods I had antibodies to were foods that I had recently eaten. However, foods that I did NOT eat—because I already knew that I was allergic to them—did not show up as allergens. I knew due to severe itching reactions that I was allergic to apples, almonds, celery, and carrots, yet the test indicated that I was not allergic to those foods. I was not eating those foods, so my body was not creating antibodies to them, but I was still definitely allergic to them! Some doctors may argue with what I am saying, but that IGG food allergy test was very misleading!

I had a variety of other allergy tests after that. One of them revealed that I was allergic to 35 different gluten (gliadin) proteins. I do react to gluten, so that was more believable. The good news is that I have healed my gut so much that most of my allergies are now healed! I can eat apples again and I enjoy them so much! This chapter covers some of the ways we self-sabotage.

Bad Habits

Autoimmune diseases can be triggered and worsened by stress. I think we all have our coping mechanisms. It might be overeating, over shopping, drinking, smoking, taking drugs or addictive medications, or unhealthy behaviors. It's a stressful life.

Yoga, meditation, loving relationships, and outdoor activities are excellent solutions to manage your stress. However, in real life, most of us only do those things when we have the time or energy, and daily responsibilities take up most of the day. Many people work indoors all day and afterwards they have to care for their family by getting dinner, doing homework, housework, etc. Post-Covid, more people than ever are telecommuting, working in their homes all day, and then doing dinner, housework, etc., in the home the rest of the day. We need more physical outlets and more time in nature to blow off some of the pent-up stress.

Smoking

I grew up surrounded by smokers and began smoking at a young age, I quit and restarted many times over the years. I quit cold turkey exactly six months before conceiving both of my children. That had to be divine intervention. For many years, I only smoked a few organic cigarettes a day. It was a hard habit to break. I was finally able to quit for good after experiencing a spiritual shift. I connected with a group of healers (and my guides) during a class and just naturally quit the next day and never smoked again. Nicotine is highly addictive and it's very difficult to give up. I'm not an expert on how to quit. I'm just sharing my experience because it's something that you may not have considered. Sometimes spiritual healing is the best healing. I found that it helped to taper down gradually, and then get in the right mindset psychologically. That way, you may not have as much of a struggle with cravings. I never had a single craving after I quit for the last time.

While I am not proud that I was dependent on cigarettes for many years, I wanted to share this struggle with my readers as a source of hope. Even though I smoked, and we all know the risks, I was still able to shrink my thyroid nodules and prevent cancer. So, no matter what your bad habits are, don't give up on yourself. There are powerful and healthy things you can do to prevent damage to your body and heal yourself.

Drinking

It is common knowledge that excess alcohol is damaging to the liver, but it can also cause damage to the heart, brain, skin, or other organs. We need our liver to function well for many purposes including blood circulation to our heart, digestion of fats, and glucose metabolism. It is in our liver where T4 is converted to T3 (the usable thyroid hormone). Our liver is an amazing organ, and it can regenerate. So, if you enjoy your drinks, just give your liver a break for a few weeks or months periodically. Nourish and support your liver with yellow and orange foods, lemon water, and herbs such as milk thistle, burdock root, yellow dock root, red clover, and chanca piedra. There are many excellent formulas to help your liver. Try to avoid developing a fatty liver by staying well-hydrated and eating a healthy anti-inflammatory diet low in fat and rich in fresh fruits and vegetables.

I drink very little now, but I drank often in the past and occasionally drank too much. I hated that feeling and I decided (several times) that I would never have another hangover. It's easier to abstain now that I feel happier and healthier. I never thought I would feel this way a few years ago, but I do. You can do it too. Sometimes, you just have to be ready.

Overeating

Like many of us, I'm a foodie. I get bored eating the same foods all the time. Food is one of the joys of life. We love to eat. We are supposed to eat to live, but I think many of us live to eat. Sometimes, we overeat when we are stressed or bored, or on special occasions. However, we can always eat lighter the next day, maybe just by having herbal teas, juiced vegetables, soup, salad, and/or fresh fruit for the whole day so your digestive system can have a break while you nourish it with fresh living enzymes. If you are tempted to overeat when you are stressed or emotional, try to wait, give it some time, go for walk or do a short workout. Before you eat or at the beginning of your meal, drink some water or herbal tea with the supplements you take with food. That will help you to feel full faster. Refer to the dietary guidelines in Chapter 11 for more helpful tips.

Overspending

It's called retail therapy. It's too easy nowadays. I'm guilty of this. I grew up poor and always felt like I didn't have enough or didn't have the things I really wanted. I have worked very hard to be able to pay my way through life and not have to rely on anyone to support me. My mother was left to support us on her own, so I learned from her that I needed to be self-reliant and work hard to make a living. She also taught me how to be a bargain hunter. I love a good deal and it really is a high, but at least it does not hurt my health. In fact, something I spend the most on is health-related stuff. That is something I do not regret. Good health is priceless, and I spend money on quality foods, supplements, and therapies to stay well.

Overworking

Working can be good. It's better than being idle. However, if you work excessive hours or experience a lot of stress or unhappiness while working, it takes a toll. Take steps to reduce your stress. For example, take breaks to stretch, eat something nutritious, take a walk, take some quality supplements, hug a family member, walk your dog, do some earthing or gardening. You get the idea. Balance is the key.

Overcoming Bad Habits

As I struggled with my health issues and the chronic stress of my technical career along with raising my boys on my own and caring for my parents, I continued to smoke a few organic cigarettes daily. I struggled with fatigue and mood swings. I was unhappy and I was afraid to gain weight when I quit smoking. After I quit for the last time, I never picked up another cigarette. I opened up about this part of my story because I'm sure there are other people that are struggling with similar issues. Some people beat themselves up and feel miserable and worry about their health.

If you have some bad habits, you should never give up on yourself. Just do the best you can to keep the bad habits to a minimum and flood your body with nutrition and self-love in the meantime to help your body repair the damage and prevent disease. For many years, I have been taking a lot of supplements and superfoods to reverse the damage from my bad habits. Apparently, it's working because I am in remission and my allergies are healed!

CHAPTER 19

Rock your Health Journey!

**"We are what we repeatedly do.
Excellence then is a habit."**
– Socrates

**"In essence, if we want to direct our lives, we must
take control of our consistent actions. It's not what
we do once in a while that shapes our lives, but what
we do consistently."**
– Tony Robbins

It is time to take action. This chapter will offer some tools and reminders to help you get healthy and rock your health journey!

I want to give you hope. I wish I had someone to guide me years ago when I was all alone trying to figure it out.

I was at my lowest point 11 years ago at 44, and now I am 55 years old, and I feel great most of the time. I am energetic and productive. I feel calmer and more resilient. I'm in a happier and more stable mood, despite this crazy world and a lifetime of emotional ups and downs. My brain clarity and memory have improved. I no longer get sick with colds, flus, or bronchitis. My heart checks out fine. My thyroid is stable and does not require a needle biopsy. I have physical pain from past injuries and when I feel inflamed, those areas flare up. I still face challenges of course, but I take them on as they come.

I was failed by one doctor after another. However, I found inspiration by researching and I was led by my intuition to find helpful books, events, people, websites, and summits. Some of those things really inspired me and helped me to improve by leaps and bounds.

I graduated from IIN in December 2012. It was a wonderful experience to study with the inspiring teachers at IIN. Taking that journey not only helped me to learn about nutrition and healing, it kept me afloat emotionally at a time when I was at my lowest.

Find what inspires you and lifts you up. Find inspiration wherever you can. Listen to a song that inspires or revs you up. Move your body. Get your blood pumping! It helps your detoxification. Dance like nobody is watching!

Your Medical Team

It is very important to assemble a great team of medical professionals.

If your doctor follows mainstream medicine only and does not have additional training in complementary medicine, try to find a practitioner that practices integrative medicine. I have been able to find very knowledgeable integrative MDs, DOs, and even an OB/GYN. I respect them and appreciate them as my medical team.

Many naturopathic doctors are excellent to work with. A naturopathic doctor typically spends two to three hours with you on your initial visit, which makes it worth spending a couple hundred dollars. If you cannot find a naturopath or functional medicine doctor near you, you can find functional medicine doctors online and schedule virtual visits.

I suggest you ask others about their medical professionals. Get referrals. If you have an integrative doctor that you respect, they are often the best people to ask for referrals to other physicians. For example, I asked my eye doctor if he knew a good cardiologist, and he got me in to see a reputable doctor by texting him for me. It doesn't hurt to ask!

You are putting your life in the hands of medical professionals, so it is very important to be selective. Do not hesitate to fire a doctor that is not providing you with good service. You don't have to tell them they are fired. Just stop going. I bet they won't call to check on you! None of mine ever did. They are far too busy. Just form the best medical team you can and try to include both allopathic and naturopathic or holistic professionals.

Health Coaching

Talking through your health journey with a compassionate advisor that takes the time to focus on you and provide you with resources and customized recommendations is so valuable. A quality certified health coach can help you to:

- Identify your top health concerns
- Review your recent medical workups and give you insights
- Clearly define and document your goals
- Document a custom diet, exercise, and supplement program

- Provide resources, recipes, tools, and eBooks to assist you
- Motivate you to stay on track and keep track of your progress

If you prefer to be your own coach:

- Make sure you always ask for a copy of your lab work (blood tests, ultrasound reports, MRI reports, etc.)
- Spend some time researching what you do not understand. Write down any questions you have and follow up with your medical team
- Follow the steps above. Discuss your medical workup with your health provider(s)
- Write down your goals, including your diet, exercise, and supplement program
- Accountability—ask someone that truly cares about you to hold you accountable
- Document your goals, including your diet, exercise, and supplement program and review it with your accountability partner. Set reminders in your calendar or phone
- Don't hesitate to get at least one coaching session to get a great head start

The Psychology of Healing

Mind over matter. Body, mind, and spirit. We are connected in so many ways that we cannot see. When you get a diagnosis, it's natural to feel concerned or frightened. However, it is best to keep a positive attitude and believe that you can heal yourself. That positive self-belief will help you to make the necessary changes to help you improve your condition.

Some people would prefer not to know what's wrong with them and there's others like me that want to know every detail. I suspect you are like me if you have read this far. I want to know everything I can about my conditions so that I can figure out how to make it better and how to prevent more problems in the future. Knowledge is power. I feel empowered when I learn.

Sometimes I slack off a little on my diet thinking that I'm doing good, that I'm healing, and I'm feeling great. Then I start experiencing symptoms and I get back on the wagon and take better care of myself. No one does everything perfectly every day. No one is perfect. We just do the best we can. Every day is a new day to take steps in the right direction.

It's like a second job having this disease. It takes time to eat right and to prepare healthy food and nutritional drinks. It takes time to take your supplements. It takes time to rest and to exercise and educate yourself. The payoff is worth it. The joy and contentment of feeling happy and energetic is priceless. If you tend to put others first, just remember they love you and want you to be healthy, and you will serve them better when you're feeling good.

Remember to believe in yourself. Your will and your resolution to heal yourself increases your odds of success.

Invest in Your Health

Do you tell yourself you cannot afford a couple hundred dollars a month for supplements and healthy foods? Don't you think it is worth a few extra bucks a month to stay healthy? Is it worth avoiding spending thousands in the long run when you become chronically ill?

Do you eat out in restaurants? You can easily spend a couple hundred dollars a month eating out. Most restaurant food has hidden fats, unhealthy and repeatedly used oils, and other hidden risks. You can prepare simple meals at home knowing what they contain while saving money you would have spent dining out.

Never Give Up

Don't ever give up no matter how old you are. We do not have to give up on feeling good when we get older.

I am happy to say that after managing Hashimoto's for about 20 years, I feel good on most days. I still deal with stiffness and pain, but I think most people in their fifties have these kinds of issues. Areas of weakness can be strengthened with exercise and improved with various therapies described in this book, such as red light therapy (described in Chapter 16).

Maintain Focus

I urge you to make a concerted effort to balance your immune system, avoid toxins, and nourish your body. If you have Hashimoto's, and if you think you can just take a daily pill and continue eating the typical American diet, I'm afraid you might end up facing some serious problems.

If you take steps to balance your health, you can prevent more serious diseases from developing. It takes some extra effort to eat healthy and feel better, but it is so worth it.

Why let this condition overtake you? Especially if giving up a few things can rev up your energy? Do you have any idea how many hours of productivity or fun you can enjoy when you get your energy back? Isn't that worth giving up a few foods? I know it's hard. If this helps, you don't have to say goodbye forever to your favorite foods. You can have a cheat day occasionally perhaps a couple times a year. However, once you get used to eating in a healthier way and once you feel better, it gets easier. If you continue to eat food that inflames your body, it is likely you will experience horrible fatigue, accelerated aging, diabetes, high cholesterol, high blood pressure, and eventually dementia. Screw that! The goal is to:

- Protect your brain
- Heal and replenish your gut
- Nourish and protect your thyroid
- Prevent cancer and keep your blood circulation healthy

Tough Love

Tough love is what I need sometimes. This is what I tell myself to stay in line or get back on track. I am well aware that I am at higher risk of diabetes and cancer because I have Hashimoto's disease and a MTHFR gene mutation. However, I choose to be proactive and take steps to detox and prevent cancer. I chose not to live in fear. If you are like me and you need some tough love, you might want to hire a health coach. If you are fortunate and you have someone in your life that will lovingly take on this role, write down your goals and the steps you plan to take to achieve them. Then, share that list with your coach or partner. Set up regularly scheduled meetings to talk about your progress, challenges, and your path forward. Being accountable to someone and having someone to talk to about your journey is very powerful.

Stay Positive

Continue to try new things at your pace and try not to get overwhelmed. Try new things with a positive outlook. Remember that it took many years to become ill, and healing doesn't happen overnight. I find it is most effective to discover the root causes of each problem and address them one by one.

Things to Remember

There is an endless amount of information available to all of us. Regardless of your current knowledge level, you can always discover new information, products, therapies, or inventions that may just result in a huge leap in your healing journey.

Key Takeaways
The top nutrient deficiencies covered in Chapter 5 include: • Vitamin D • Vitamin B12 • Selenium • Zinc • Magnesium • Iron/ferritin • Thiamine (Vitamin B1)
The most common underlying causes of adrenal fatigue (covered in Chapter 5) include: • Chronic sleep deprivation • Too much caffeine • Lack of exercise • Chronic stress and shock • Not enough vitamins and minerals • Chronic pain and inflammation • Underlying infection
Make sure you have addressed any infections and have detoxed from heavy metals (covered in Chapter 6).
Consider taking Modified Citrus Pectin regularly to prevent aging and the disease process.

Tips for Reducing Toxin Exposure

Here is a general list of how you can avoid toxins:

- Avoid processed foods
- Avoid non-organic foods, at least those in the dirty dozen
- Avoid conventionally raised meat or dairy (organic and grass fed is better)
- Avoid farm-raised fish or large fish
- Avoid high-fructose corn syrup

- Avoid artificial sweeteners. Stevia and monk fruit are safe and taste great
- Avoid health and beauty products that have long lists of ingredients including chemicals you cannot pronounce
- If you own a home, consider a whole-house water filtration system
- Use chemical free products at home for cleaning, air freshening, etc.
- Determine if you live near a nuclear plant, fracking well or coal-burning plant
- If you have mercury fillings, consult with a dentist skilled in safe replacement
- Consider testing the water and air in your home for toxins and mold

Stress Reduction Tips

Remember that stress is a major trigger of autoimmune symptoms. Here are some tips to reduce stress:

- Remember to breathe deeply. Use the 4:7:8 breathing technique (from Chapter 17).
- Do your best to delegate. Don't take everything on in the house yourself. If your children are young, give them small chores to get them used to having a "job." They have tons of energy. Let them help.
- Laughter boosts your oxytocin levels. This helps to counteract the stress hormone, cortisol. Watch or listen to funny shows as you get things done. Call a friend for some laughs, especially the sarcastic ones. It's fun to laugh at the craziness of life!
- Hug your family and friends often, as affection boosts your oxytocin levels.
- Be mindful of listening to positive programs and avoid programs with fear, violence, and negativity.

- Schedule time to exercise daily to avoid stiffness and injury. Yoga, Pilates, low-impact cardio, upper body strengthening, and dancing are excellent choices to reduce stress and maintain strength and flexibility.
- Schedule time to organize and do bills regularly so things don't pile up.
- Spend time outside and enjoy fresh air, walks, and the beauty of nature.
- Get things off your chest by writing them in a journal or talking with trusted confidants.

Conclusion

Remember to love yourself.

Loving yourself is a primary key to the next breakthrough that you are looking for.

Say you are going to exercise 15 mins every day. Understand that when you procrastinate, it contributes to a lack of trust or belief in yourself. If we really love ourselves every single day, we'll find the time to do the things that are important for our own physical, mental, and spiritual health.

Put time and energy into what YOU love.

Focus on getting the good stuff in. Try to get protein, fiber, healthy fat, and antioxidants at every meal. Eat plenty of vegetables. Stay away from carbs, grains, alcohol, sugar, gluten, fried foods, all the bad stuff!

Get outside into the sunshine regularly, especially in the morning sun. It's good for your eyes and a great way to start the day.

Remember what you have learned and don't put this book down and forget about it. I don't want the time you spent reading this book to be futile. Keep the momentum you are feeling. Mark the pages that resonate with you with post-it notes to remind you of the steps you want to take to get better.

Discuss what you have read with your loved ones. Start a journal and write down what you plan to do to improve your health.

This journey can be lonely. Make sure you have some support along the way even if it's from a stranger. There are many of us struggling with this.

Love yourself. Be patient with yourself. This is not easy. YOU ARE WORTH IT.

Acknowledgments

David Wolfe

A very special thank you to David Wolfe. Although I have conducted cancer and nutritional research since I was 18 years old, David taught me a lot of new information about the science of healing, superfoods, and super herbs. He was one of my teachers at the Institute for Integrative Medicine (IIN). He stimulated my intellect as he described the power of superfoods such as goji berries, medicinal herbs, and mushrooms (which are also herbs). He amused me with his humor and sarcasm which made it more fun to learn. He has a cheeky grin and inner happiness that shines through while he reveals the truth about incredible foods, herbs, and natural medicines that are not generally known.

I honestly do not know if I would have been able to shrink my thyroid nodules without him. His enthusiasm and zest for the best herbs ever, best foods ever, and best water ever is absolutely "infectious" in a GREAT way. David teaches the next level in super nutrition. He helped to bring many "superfoods" to the mainstream market, including hemp seed, chia seed, goji berries, and medicinal mushrooms. I had the pleasure to meet him in person in Nashville in 2021. I was at my highest weight after having gained additional pounds during the pandemic which was compounded by the grief of losing my mother and having major shoulder surgery. He gave me a big hug and I gave him a gift of cinnamon frankincense pain cream and sacred skin oil that I made. I look forward to seeing him again and handing him a copy of this book!

The Institute for Integrative Nutrition

I'd also like to thank all my teachers along the way. I began studying natural health in the 1990s and I never stopped. It started with paper newsletters from Dr. Julian Whittaker, and I'll never forget his newsletter about Down's syndrome and the effectiveness of mega doses of vitamins. I joined the Institute for Integrative Nutrition in 2012 which was founded and led by Joshua Rosenthal. Thank you, Joshua, for teaching with so much love, compassion, and humor. I miss your lectures. I greatly appreciate the education I received at IIN. I was exposed to a whole new group of amazing leaders in the nutritional and medical world. Some of my favorites include Mark Hyman, Joel Fuhrman, Barry Sears, David Perlmutter, Daniel Amen, Sally Fallon, and Andrea Beaman. I also gained new insights from teachers I had already followed such as Christine Northrup, William Davis, Dr. Andrew Weil, and Bernie Siegel.

My Special Boys

Thank you to my two very special sons, Adam, and Adrian. Throughout all the years that I struggled there were many times I was too exhausted to make dinner or too drained to spend quality time with them. They were always loving and understanding and gave me pure love, hugs, and laughter every single day. When I was spending many days on my bed, barely getting up, many times with foot pain, back pain, ankle injuries, or just plain exhaustion, they would come in my room throughout the day to hug me and talk to me. They build me up. The love between all three of us is strong and beautiful.

They know my heart better than anyone and they have far exceeded any expectations that I could ever have had as far as how a parent-child relationship can be. I felt a little distant from my parents growing up and part of that was generational. However, religion also factored in and created a divide. With my children, communication and respect have always been present. They are respectful, kind, warm, and humorous. I could never have predicted or planned the outcome. They are just my heart. Forever.

Karin Hansen – Friend and Designer

Thank you, Karin, my soul sister, for always supporting me throughout my healing journey and this journey of life. Thank you for always believing in me and supporting my dreams. Karin designed the cover of this book, which came out beautifully, and was exactly what I had in mind. She is an incredibly talented visual and creative designer. She has created my business logos, business cards, flyers, brochures, and the labels for all of my Indigo Healing Oils products. Although physical distance separates us now, we are never far apart in spirit. We will continue to support and inspire each other through good times and bad, anything that comes our way.

Halina Okla – Friend and Anti-Aging Enthusiast

Thank you Halina, my soul sister, for always being a seeker and experimentalist in the world of anti-aging and healing. Halina is one of few people in my life that presents me with new healing modalities before I hear about them. She is always finding new treatments and devices to stay young, vital, and moving. Now in her early seventies, she is still constantly on the move, still working, and traveling often. She is an inspiration to me. She makes her own colloidal silver. She collects her own fresh spring water. We have done hyperbaric oxygen therapy together, intravenous vitamin therapy, healing waters, and mushroom hunting for medicinal tree mushrooms. We love going salsa dancing together, and listening to merengue, bachata, and salsa music. We also love animals, and we frequent farms together. We attend expos and conferences on the latest in natural health, beauty, and spirituality whenever we can. We are both currently experimenting with scalar energy healing. She looks much younger than her years. We are both inspired to help others to heal, and each other. I look forward to many more adventures with Halina. My girl Halina, young at heart forever! May you live to be 150 years young!

About the Author

Julie Diaz is a Certified Integrative Health Coach, Technical Writer, Author, and Speaker. She was diagnosed with Hashimoto's autoimmune disease in 2012 after more than 10 years of seeking help from various doctors. Once properly diagnosed, she devised her own holistic regimen, and successfully shrank two thyroid nodules within two months using the natural medicine program she created. She was able to avoid thyroid removal surgery and achieve remission, while reclaiming her energy, happiness, and productivity.

Julie draws inspiration from nature and believes tapping into your higher self helps to put you on a path to greater balance, joy, and growth. She enjoys reading non-fiction, dancing, painting, making crystal jewelry, and creating natural remedies from herbs and essential oils. Julie is an avid health researcher and is passionate about helping others to heal. She investigates the root causes of illness and is always learning about the latest and greatest (and even historically proven) ways to heal and prevent disease with diet, lifestyle, vitamins, herbs, nutraceuticals, and even scalar frequencies.

Julie lives in New Jersey with her family. When not writing and researching, she spends her time walking in nature, gardening, watching movies, listening to music, attending concerts, and traveling. Julie holds degrees in Computer Science and Psychology, and multiple certifications in health coaching, nutrition, aromatherapy, and herbology.

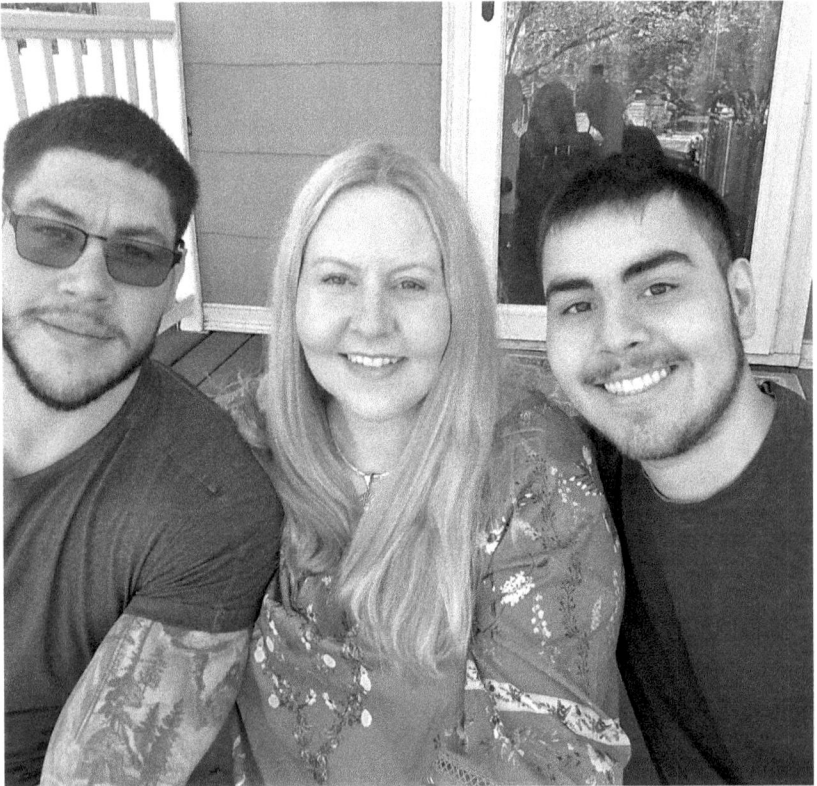

References

[1] https://www.naturalnews.com/043264_thyroid_nodules_nutrition_pharmaceutical_medicine.html

[2] https://autoimmune.org/insight-conversations-with-thought-leaders/

[3] https://pubmed.ncbi.nlm.nih.gov/3066320/#:~:text=An%20autoimmune%20cause%20accounts%20for%20approximately%2090%25,of%20adult%20hypothyroidism%2C%20mostly%20due%20to%20Hashimoto%27s%20disease.

[4] https://www.ncbi.nlm.nih.gov/pmc/articles/PMC3318917/

[5] https://www.thyroid.org/media-main/press-room/

[6] https://pubmed.ncbi.nlm.nih.gov/28536577/

[7] https://www.sernova.com/press/release/?id=355

[8] https://theconversation.com/will-the-new-toxic-chemical-safety-law-protect-us-60769

[9] https://www.gao.gov/assets/gao-13-249.pdf

[10] https://thyroidpharmacist.com/articles/genes-associated-hashimotos/

[11] https://pubmed.ncbi.nlm.nih.gov/24678255/

[12] https://drjockers.com/glyphosate-what-is-it-testing-and-detox-strategies/

[13] https://www.webmd.com/a-to-z-guides/what-is-a-functional-medicine-doctor#:~:text=They%20consider%20factors%20like%20diet%2C%20genetics%2C%20hormonal%20changes%2C,that%20aren%27t%20e-asily%20managed%20by%20conventional%20medical%20techniques.

14 https://www.thyroid.org/wp-content/uploads/patients/brochures/Postpartum_Thyroiditis_brochure.pdf

15 https://academic.oup.com/jcem/article/92/4/1263/2596911

16 https://nyulangone.org/conditions/thyroid-nodules-cancers/types

17 https://www.thyroid.org/goiter/

18 https://www.hopkinsmedicine.org/health/conditions-and-diseases/thyroid-nodules-when-to-worry

19 https://www.cancer.org/research/cancer-facts-statistics.html

20 https://thyroidpharmacist.com/articles/top-things-know-thyroid-cancer/

21 https://www.cancer.org/cancer/thyroid-cancer/about/key-statistics.html

22 https://pubmed.ncbi.nlm.nih.gov/2408737/

23 https://www.mayoclinic.org/tests-procedures/thyroidectomy/about/pac-20385195

24 https://www.umms.org/ummc/health-services/surgery/endocrine-surgery/conditions/thyroid-gland/risks

25 https://rdcu.be/c6aB3

26 https://www.thyroid.org/patient-thyroid-information/ct-for-patients/volume-issue-december/vol-8-issue-12-p-3-4/

27 https://pubmed.ncbi.nlm.nih.gov/3066320/

28 https://thyroidpharmacist.com/articles/is-your-medication-gluten-free/

29 https://thyroidpharmacist.com/articles/9-medications-toxic-thyroid/

30 https://pubmed.ncbi.nlm.nih.gov/7476598/

31 https://www.sciencedaily.com/releases/1999/09/990910080344.htm

32 https://pubmed.ncbi.nlm.nih.gov/34537272/

33 https://www.singlecare.com/blog/most-prescribed-drugs-2021/

34 https://thyroidpharmacist.com/articles/top-10-thyroid-tests/

35 https://www.ncbi.nlm.nih.gov/pmc/articles/PMC6008310/

36 https://www.researchgate.net/publication/275664957_The_role_of_Epstein-Barr_virus_infection_in_the_development_of_autoimmune_thyroid_diseases

37 https://www.ncbi.nlm.nih.gov/pmc/articles/PMC6025560/

38 https://en.wikipedia.org/wiki/Gastroparesis

39 https://www.nih.gov/news-events/nih-research-matters/gut-microbe-drives-autoimmunity

40 https://journals.lww.com/jcge/abstract/1998/06000/helicobacter_pylori_infection_is_markedly.8.aspx

References

41 https://journals.sagepub.com/doi/pdf/10.5698/1535-7511-14.s2.29

42 https://www.ncbi.nlm.nih.gov/pmc/articles/PMC6237250/

43 https://autoimmune.org/lyme-disease-and-the-autoimmune-connection/#:~:text=Post%2DTreatment%20Lyme%20Disease%20Syndrome%20and%20Autoimmune%20Diseases&text=Additionally%-2C%20some%20patients%20may%20develop,thyroid%20disease%2C%20and%20autoimmune%20neuropathy.

44 https://entomologytoday.org/2021/01/22/mapping-lyme-cdc-reveals-distribution-of-lyme-disease-causing-bacteria-county-ticks/

45 https://www.youtube.com/watch?v=1w0_kazbb_U

46 https://www.dovepress.com/getfile.php?fileID=5448

47 https://www.ncbi.nlm.nih.gov/pmc/articles/PMC3988285/

48 https://pubmed.ncbi.nlm.nih.gov/30742953/

49 https://pubmed.ncbi.nlm.nih.gov/8153237/

50 https://www.nature.com/articles/s41415-019-0331-6#:~:text=It%20is%20estimated%20that%20two-thirds%20of%20dental%20mercury,can%20undergo%20conversion%20to%20methylmercury%20by%20aquatic%20microorganisms.

51 https://www.cdc.gov/flu/prevent/thimerosal.htm

52 https://www.nejm.org/doi/full/10.1056/NEJMp078187

53 https://pubmed.ncbi.nlm.nih.gov/29895363/

54 https://www.cdc.gov/vaccinesafety/concerns/thimerosal/index.html

55 https://pubmed.ncbi.nlm.nih.gov/22099156/

56 https://www.ncbi.nlm.nih.gov/pmc/articles/PMC5256113/

57 https://pubmed.ncbi.nlm.nih.gov/23609067/

58 https://pubmed.ncbi.nlm.nih.gov/36184718/

59 https://pubmed.ncbi.nlm.nih.gov/21157018/

60 https://www.spandidos-publications.com/10.3892/mmr.2017.6381#:~:text=Several%20studies%20demonstrated%20that%20exposure,infectious%20disease%2C%20autoimmunity%20or%20cancer.

61 https://pubmed.ncbi.nlm.nih.gov/19540334/

62 https://www.iowadnr.gov/portals/idnr/uploads/water/standards/files/k_arsenic.pdf

63 https://greenmedinfo.com/article/inorganic-arsenic-contents-rice-based-infant-foods-spain-uk-china-and-usa

64 https://nutritionfacts.org/blog/why-was-chicken-the-primary-source-of-arsenic-exposure-in-children/

65 https://pubmed.ncbi.nlm.nih.gov/18029502/

66 https://pubmed.ncbi.nlm.nih.gov/36858772/

67 https://en.wikipedia.org/wiki/Perchlorate

68 https://www.ncbi.nlm.nih.gov/pmc/articles/PMC4137763/

69 https://www.ncbi.nlm.nih.gov/pmc/articles/PMC1940071/

70 https://www.ncbi.nlm.nih.gov/pmc/articles/PMC2935336/

71 https://pubmed.ncbi.nlm.nih.gov/21061092/

72 https://thyroidnation.com/whiplash-hashimotos-trigger-swan-dive/

73 https://www.ncbi.nlm.nih.gov/pmc/articles/PMC6025560/

74 https://pubmed.ncbi.nlm.nih.gov/32166585/

76 https://www.webmd.com/diet/health-benefits-chaga-tea

77 https://ldnresearchtrust.org/how-low-dose-naltrexone-works

78 https://ldnresearchtrust.org/conditions

79 http://lowdosenaltrexone.org/faq.html#What_diseases_has_it_been_useful_for

80 https://ldnresearchtrust.org/

81 https://www.ldnscience.org/ldn/how-does-ldn-work

82 https://www.epa.gov/mercury/what-do-if-mercury-thermometer-breaks

83 https://www.ncbi.nlm.nih.gov/pmc/articles/PMC7129276/

84 https://pubmed.ncbi.nlm.nih.gov/24238833/

85 https://www.ncbi.nlm.nih.gov/pmc/articles/PMC5256113/

86 https://www.ewg.org/

87 https://pubmed.ncbi.nlm.nih.gov/35956821/

88 https://pubmed.ncbi.nlm.nih.gov/16835878/

89 https://www.atsdr.cdc.gov/csem/arsenic/patient_instructions.html

90 https://greenmedinfo.com/article/curcumin-reduces-arsenic-induced-dna-damage-human-subjects

91 https://www.dentistrytoday.com/eu-commission-bans-use-of-dental-amalgam-from-2025/

92 https://www.ncbi.nlm.nih.gov/pmc/articles/PMC6704025/

93 https://iaomt.org/resources/dental-mercury-facts/mercury-poisoning-symptoms-dental-amalgam/

94 https://draxe.com/nutrition/n-acetyl-cysteine-nac-supplement-benefits/

95 https://www.ncbi.nlm.nih.gov/pmc/articles/PMC8229678/

References

96 https://www.npr.org/sections/thesalt/2015/12/09/459061317/a-protein-in-the-gut-may-explain-why-some-cant-stomach-gluten#:~:text=It%20turns%20out%20that%20gluten,to%20high%20levels%20of%20it

97 https://link.springer.com/article/10.1007/s12016-011-8291-x

98 https://pubmed.ncbi.nlm.nih.gov/24483336/

99 https://www.fda.gov/food/agricultural-biotechnology/how-gmos-are-regulated-united-states

100 https://www.ams.usda.gov/rules-regulations/be/consumers

101 https://www.centerforfoodsafety.org/issues/311/ge-foods/about-ge-foods#:~:text=It%20has%20been%20estimated%20that,condiments%20%E2%80%93%20contain%20genetically%20engineered%20ingredients.

102 https://pubmed.ncbi.nlm.nih.gov/22337346/

103 https://www.ewg.org/take-action

104 https://pubmed.ncbi.nlm.nih.gov/27307072/

105 https://www.ncbi.nlm.nih.gov/pmc/articles/PMC2879161/

106 https://ipen.org/news/new-study-finds-lead-levels-majority-paints-exceed-chinese-regulation-and-should-not-be-store

107 https://thetruthaboutcancer.com/what-is-an-elimination-diet/

108 https://www.ncbi.nlm.nih.gov/pmc/articles/PMC8313054/

109 https://pubmed.ncbi.nlm.nih.gov/29511601/

110 https://pubmed.ncbi.nlm.nih.gov/30060266/

111 https://www.ewg.org/foodnews/full-list.php

112 https://thyroidpharmacist.com/articles/soy-and-hashimotos/

113 https://www.hindawi.com/journals/jdr/2013/390534/

114 https://thyroidpharmacist.com/articles/hashimotos-blood-sugar-and-diabetes/

115 https://www.hindawi.com/journals/ije/2016/9132052/

116 https://pubmed.ncbi.nlm.nih.gov/16380698/

117 https://link.springer.com/article/10.1007/s13679-022-00481-1

118 https://pubmed.ncbi.nlm.nih.gov/37697017/

119 https://www.webmd.com/diet/ss/slideshow-all-about-the-paleo-diet

120 https://pubmed.ncbi.nlm.nih.gov/36598468/

121 https://www.webmd.com/diet/what-to-know-about-the-aip-diet

122 https://www.webmd.com/ibd-crohns-disease/crohns-disease/specific-carbohydrate-diet-overview

[123] http://www.greenmedinfo.com/blog/iodine-fuel-fire-hashimoto-s

[124] https://www.mayoclinic.org/diseases-conditions/hypothyroidism/expert-answers/hypothyroidism-iodine/faq-20057929

[125] https://www.thyroid.org/american-thyroid-association-ata-issues-statement-on-the-potential-risks-of-excess-iodine-ingestion-and-exposure/

[126] https://pubmed.ncbi.nlm.nih.gov/3722332/

[127] https://www.ncbi.nlm.nih.gov/pmc/articles/PMC4139880/

[128] https://www.townsendletter.com/AugSept2005/gabyiodine0805.htm

[129] https://www.tandfonline.com/doi/abs/10.3109/09637486.2016.1144717

[130] https://thyroidpharmacist.com/articles/iodine-hashimotos/

[131] https://greenmedinfo.com/blog/iodine-fuel-fire-hashimoto-s

[132] https://www.mdpi.com/2072-6643/2/6/611

[133] https://pubmed.ncbi.nlm.nih.gov/26305620/

[134] https://academic.oup.com/jcem/article/92/4/1263/2596911

[135] https://pubmed.ncbi.nlm.nih.gov/26404370/

[136] https://pubmed.ncbi.nlm.nih.gov/26675817/

[137] https://pubmed.ncbi.nlm.nih.gov/23379830/

[138] https://pubmed.ncbi.nlm.nih.gov/24351023/

[139] https://pubmed.ncbi.nlm.nih.gov/25758370/

[140] https://www.ncbi.nlm.nih.gov/books/NBK441912/

[141] https://www.acam.org/page/Searches

[142] https://pubmed.ncbi.nlm.nih.gov/21310306/

[143] https://www.wbur.org/hereandnow/2019/01/28/mushrooms-fungi-disease-bees

[144] https://www.bbc.com/future/article/20190314-the-unexpected-magic-of-mushrooms

[145] https://www.ncbi.nlm.nih.gov/pmc/articles/PMC8409941/

[146] https://www.ncbi.nlm.nih.gov/pmc/articles/PMC8876642/

[147] https://www.ncbi.nlm.nih.gov/pmc/articles/PMC8409941/

[148] https://www.ncbi.nlm.nih.gov/pmc/articles/PMC4946216/

[149] https://pubmed.ncbi.nlm.nih.gov/18203281/

[150] https://www.ncbi.nlm.nih.gov/pmc/articles/PMC8124789/

[151] https://www.ncbi.nlm.nih.gov/pmc/articles/PMC5302426/

[152] https://pubmed.ncbi.nlm.nih.gov/17895634/

[153] https://pubmed.ncbi.nlm.nih.gov/37233262/

[154] https://pubmed.ncbi.nlm.nih.gov/23557368/

[155] https://pubmed.ncbi.nlm.nih.gov/26853960/

[156] https://pubmed.ncbi.nlm.nih.gov/27481156/

[157] https://pubmed.ncbi.nlm.nih.gov/23510212/

[158] https://pubmed.ncbi.nlm.nih.gov/34169530/

[159] https://pubmed.ncbi.nlm.nih.gov/35877305/

[160] https://pubmed.ncbi.nlm.nih.gov/29238712/

[161] https://medicinalherbals.net/agaricus-blazei-murill/

[162] https://www.hindawi.com/journals/jtr/2013/424163/#results

[163] https://www.ncbi.nlm.nih.gov/pmc/articles/PMC5331475/

[164] https://pubmed.ncbi.nlm.nih.gov/29053604/

[165] https://nationalmenopauseassociation.com/pcos-menopause-inositol/

[166] https://pubmed.ncbi.nlm.nih.gov/20811299/

[167] https://pubmed.ncbi.nlm.nih.gov/23682780/

[168] https://www.ncbi.nlm.nih.gov/pmc/articles/PMC4263715/

[169] https://pubmed.ncbi.nlm.nih.gov/25869292/

[170] https://www.ncbi.nlm.nih.gov/pmc/articles/PMC8696197/

[171] https://draxe.com/nutrition/berberine/

[172] https://pubmed.ncbi.nlm.nih.gov/15913551/

[173] https://pubmed.ncbi.nlm.nih.gov/29480200/

[174] https://pubmed.ncbi.nlm.nih.gov/7809573/

[175] https://pubmed.ncbi.nlm.nih.gov/18222135/

[176] https://pubmed.ncbi.nlm.nih.gov/23957171/

[177] https://pubmed.ncbi.nlm.nih.gov/17907184/

[178] https://pubmed.ncbi.nlm.nih.gov/20036139/

[179] http://orthomolecular.org/resources/omns/v19n27.shtml

[180] https://pubmed.ncbi.nlm.nih.gov/27852303/

[181] https://www.sciencedaily.com/releases/2016/05/160520142903.htm

[182] https://www.ewg.org/childrenshealth/monsanto-weedkiller-still-contaminates-foods-marketed-to-children?utm_source=newsletter&utm_campaign=9999Recapture3&utm_medium=email&emci=bc2e9fec-bbdb-ec11-b656-281878b8c32f&emdi=738b5265-0280-ed11-9d7a-000d3a9eb913&ceid=3806028

[183] https://www.jointhemany.com/

[184] https://pubmed.ncbi.nlm.nih.gov/21974805/

185 https://pubmed.ncbi.nlm.nih.gov/15375548/

186 https://www.ncbi.nlm.nih.gov/pmc/articles/PMC1950436/

187 https://pubmed.ncbi.nlm.nih.gov/34462562/

188 https://pubmed.ncbi.nlm.nih.gov/12488479/

189 https://ascopubs.org/doi/abs/10.1200/JCO.2023.41.6_suppl.162

190 https://www.ncbi.nlm.nih.gov/pmc/articles/PMC2782490/

191 https://www.dogcancerblog.com/articles/full-spectrum-cancer-care/supplements/modified-citrus-pectin-dogs/

192 https://www.ncbi.nlm.nih.gov/pmc/articles/PMC1950436/

193 https://pubmed.ncbi.nlm.nih.gov/18219211/

194 https://pubmed.ncbi.nlm.nih.gov/18616067/

195 https://pubmed.ncbi.nlm.nih.gov/33484445/

196 https://pubmed.ncbi.nlm.nih.gov/25794149/

197 https://www.ncbi.nlm.nih.gov/pmc/articles/PMC6277462/

198 https://pubmed.ncbi.nlm.nih.gov/22147334/

199 https://pubmed.ncbi.nlm.nih.gov/21315510/

200 https://pubmed.ncbi.nlm.nih.gov/36972873/

201 https://supplements.selfdecode.com/blog/zeolite-benefits/

202 https://www.yeastinfectionadvisor.com/support-files/powdered-zeolite-versus-liquids.pdf

203 https://pubmed.ncbi.nlm.nih.gov/26084226/

204 https://gerson.org/

205 https://pubmed.ncbi.nlm.nih.gov/32152852/

206 https://pubmed.ncbi.nlm.nih.gov/28615356/

207 https://www.ncbi.nlm.nih.gov/pmc/articles/PMC6472148/

208 https://pubmed.ncbi.nlm.nih.gov/25842380/

209 https://link.springer.com/article/10.1007/s10787-018-0531-8

210 https://www.lifeextension.com/magazine/2009/ss/powerful-advances-in-natural-cancer-prevention

211 https://pubmed.ncbi.nlm.nih.gov/17212569/

212 https://chemocare.com/chemotherapy/side-effects/depression-and-chemotherapy.aspx

213 https://www.healthline.com/health/confusion-after-chemotherapy#causes

214 https://www.youtube.com/watch?v=6scWQ2sYNvI

215 https://www.burzynskiclinic.com/dr-stanislaw-r-burzynski/

References

216 https://jeffreydachmd.com/wp-content/uploads/2013/07/Clinical_Guide_ Vitamin_C_Lendon_Smith_2006.pdf

217 https://en.wikipedia.org/wiki/Linus_Pauling

218 https://greenmedinfo.com/blog/linus-pauling-heart-disease-prevention-vitamin-c

219 https://pubmed.ncbi.nlm.nih.gov/34717701/

220 https://www.sciencedaily.com/releases/2014/02/140210135908.htm

221 https://www.drugwatch.com/vioxx/

222 http://www.doctoryourself.com/strategies.html

223 https://media.mercola.com/ImageServer/Public/2021/October/PDF/ vitamin-d-to-prevent-tumor-death-pdf.pdf

224 https://mthfrsupport.com/

225 https://thyroidpharmacist.com/articles/mthfr-hashimotos-and-nutrients/

226 https://www.discovermagazine.com/the-sciences/ dna-is-not-destiny-the-new-science-of-epigenetics

227 https://www.drbenlynch.com/

228 https://drjockers.com/red-light-therapy/

229 https://pubmed.ncbi.nlm.nih.gov/20662037/

230 https://pubmed.ncbi.nlm.nih.gov/21172691/

231 https://pubmed.ncbi.nlm.nih.gov/24049929/

232 https://pubmed.ncbi.nlm.nih.gov/35966907/

233 https://pubmed.ncbi.nlm.nih.gov/23970445/

234 https://pubmed.ncbi.nlm.nih.gov/31151332/

235 https://pubmed.ncbi.nlm.nih.gov/26858986/

236 https://www.lifeextension.com/protocols/metabolic-health/hypothyroidism

237 https://pubmed.ncbi.nlm.nih.gov/27536198/

238 https://www.ncbi.nlm.nih.gov/pmc/articles/PMC6985662/#cpr12712-bib-0007

239 https://pubmed.ncbi.nlm.nih.gov/20841611/

240 https://pubmed.ncbi.nlm.nih.gov/27333945/

241 https://pubmed.ncbi.nlm.nih.gov/23183379/

242 https://www.sernova.com/press/release/?id=355

243 https://pubmed.ncbi.nlm.nih.gov/35778957/

244 https://pubmed.ncbi.nlm.nih.gov/28792455/

245 https://lifestylemedicine.org/articles/ benefits-plant-based-nutrition-autoimmune-disease/

[246] https://pubmed.ncbi.nlm.nih.gov/32172066/

[247] https://pubmed.ncbi.nlm.nih.gov/6307932/

[248] https://www.ncbi.nlm.nih.gov/pmc/articles/PMC3158557/

[249] https://superfoodly.com/orac-values/

Index

Index

371

Index

– H –

– N –

Index

Index

www.ingramcontent.com/pod-product-compliance
Lightning Source LLC
Chambersburg PA
CBHW052107030426
42335CB00025B/2875